Anesthesia and emergency

HALA GOMA

PROFESSOR OF ANESTHESIA CAIRO UNIVERSITY

Table of contents

Introduction

Patient may needs anesthesia in elective surgery and emergency surgery. In elective surgery there is time for proper preparation of the patient as full history, full investigations, and may be an preparatory operation for major operation such carotid end arterectomy before coronary bypass grafting. Anesthetist may be faced by an urgent operation which increased risk for morbidity and mortality. Such operations as obstetric bleeding, postoperative bleeding, another emergency situation as perioperative myocardial infarction, anesthesia during septicemia or septic shock .intraoperative emergency as anaphylaxis or local anesthetic toxicity .in this book I discussed these emergency situations and how to prepare the patient and so decrease the intraoperative and postoperative mortality.

What are the anesthetic emergency?

- Hemorrhage

1. Obstetric hemorrhage

   Hemorrhage (APH, PPH)

2. Surgical bleeding

- Pulmonary Embolism

- Amniotic Fluid Embolism.

- Cardiac (Valvular HD)

- Sepsis

- Respiratory emergency

- **Myocardial Infarction**
- **Anaphylaxis.**
- **Local Anesthetic Toxicity.**

Maternal hemorrhage:

Hemorrhage is the major cause of maternal collapse in

Labor ward

Postpartum Hemorrhage

ETIOLOGY

- Retained placenta

- Placenta Accreta

- Uterine atony

- Vaginal and cervical laceration

- DIC, AFE

- Factor disorder

- Uterine rupture / Uterine inversio

Class	Acute Blood Loss	% Lost
1	900cc	15
2	1200-1500cc	20-25

3	1800-2100cc	30-35
4	2400cc	40

ASSESSMENT OF BLOOD LOSS AFTER DELIVERY

- Difficult

- Mostly Visual estimation (So, Subjective & Inaccurate)

- Underestimation is likely

- Clinical picture -Misleading

- Our Mothers-Malnourished, Anemic, Small built, Less blood volume

SYMPTOMS & SIGNS

Modified Early Warning Scoring System   (MEWS)

MEWS calculated from 5 physiological

   variables

- **Mental response**

- Pulse rate

- Systolic BP

- Respiratory rate

- Temperature

Modified Early Warning Scoring System
(MEWS)

Respiratory rate of ≥25 or <10 breaths per minute.
- Arterial systolic blood pressure of <90mmHg.

- Heart rate of ≥110 or <55 beats per minute.

- Not fully alert and orientated.

- Oxygen saturation of <90 per cent.

- Urine output over the last four hours of <100ml

- Respiratory rate ≥35 breaths per minute or a heart rate ≥140 beats per minute.

Clinical Features of Shock

Risk factors for postoperative bleeding

- Liver or kidney disease,

- Bleeding disorder, such as hemophilia

- Medicines such as aspirin.

- Vitamin or herbal supplements that affect blood clotting, such as vitamin E, ginkgo, ginseng, or feverfew

<u>Classification of postoperative bleeding</u>

Primary bleeding –
- Bleeding that occurs within the intra-operative period.
- This should be resolved during the operation, the patient monitored closely post-operatively.

Reactive bleeding

It occurs within 24 hours of operation.

Most cases of reactive hemorrhage are from a ligature that slips or a missed vessel.

These vessels can be missed intraoperatively due to intraoperative hypotension and vasoconstriction,

Secondary bleeding
- It occurs 7-10 days post-operatively.
- Secondary hemorrhage is often due to erosion of a vessel from spreading infection.
- Secondary hemorrhage is most often seen when a heavily contaminated wound is closed primarily.

<u>High risk surgical procedures for postoperative bleeding</u>

a. **Thyroidectomy** or **para thyroidectomy** hemorrhage Post-operative bleeding can have catastrophic consequences and **airway obstruction** is likely to be The primary sign of haemorrhage

b. **Inferior Epigastric Artery Injury** It is susceptible to injury from **laparoscopic ports.**

c. Retroperitoneal Bleeding Post-Angiography

Differential diagnosis of post-operative hypotension

Hypovolemia

(1) The blood which is lost at the operation has not been replaced

(2) The fluid which is lost into his sequestrated gut has not been replaced.

(3) Deep anesthesia, respiration is depressed, leading to hypoxemia and hypotension.

(4) Administration of large doses of opioids, such as morphine or pethidine.

(5) High subarachnoid (spinal) anesthetic (A 7.4).

(6) Septicemia

(7) The gut may have been roughly handled.

(8) The patient may be roughly handled on a trolley.

	Class I	Class II	Class III	Class IV
Blood Loss (ml)	<750ml	750-1500ml	1500-2000	>2000
Blood Loss (%)	<15%	15-30%	30-40%	>40%
Heart Rate	<100	100-120	120-140	>140
Blood Pressure	Normal	Normal	Decreased	Decreased
Respiratory Rate	14-20	20-30	30-40	>40
Urine Output (mL/hr)	>30	20-30	5-20	<5

Table 1: Classification of Hemorrhagic Shock

Clinical picture of hemorrhagic shock

- Fast pulse

- Pallor

- Abdominal distension

- Bright red blood from a drain incision

- If two units of blood do not restore his blood pressure, consider reopening the wound to control the bleeding.

- If, after a stomach operation, after aspiration of fresh blood from the nasogastric tube the bleeding is from the anastomosis in the stomach. If the blood pressure is only a little depressed, perform gastric lavage every half hour with iced water containing 8 mg of noradrenalin 200 ml.

- If more than 3 units of blood to maintain his blood pressure above 100 mm is required, and there is aspirating fresh blood an hour later, exploration of the patients is must.

- If the bleeding from gut some days after the operation, the blood may be coming from a stress ulcer, or from a pre-existing duodenal ulcer.

- Monitor the pulse, blood pressure, and urine output. Keep a good drip going, and measure hematocrit 3-hourly.

- Have at least two units of blood cross-matched.

- Irrigate the stomach with iced saline or tap water containing noradrenalin 8 mg in 200 ml every half hour.

- **Blood tests** prothromin concentration , INR ,platelets, clotting time

- Endoscopy and angiography may be used to find the source of your bleeding, or to control it.

Management of Hemorrhage

- ■ **RESUSITATION OF Hemorrhagic Shock**

- ■ **Cardiac Arrest -(CPR)**

RESUSITATION OF Hemorrhagic Shock

- o **Oxygen by mask 10 liter/min. to keep O2 saturation > 94%**

- o **1st IV Line: Ringer Lactate**

- o **Sample blood; CBC, fibrinogen, PT/PTT, platelets, and order 4u PRBC**

- o **Urinary Foley catheter**

- Get **Obstetrician, Anesthesiologist, surgeon, Interventional Radiology, Intensives**, and Hematologist**.

Management of Obstetrical Hemorrhage.

- LR or NS replaces blood loss at 3:1

- Volume expander 1:1 (albumin, hetastarch, dextran)

- Anticipate Disseminated Intravascular Coagulopathy (DIC)

- Verify complete removal of placenta, may need ultrasound

- Inspect for bleeding

- -episiotomy, laceration, hematomas, inversion, rupture
- Emperic transfusion

- -2 u PRBC; FFP 1-2 u/4-5 u PRBC
- Cryo 10 u,
- Uncrossed (O neg.) PRBC – For emergency
- Warm all blood products and I.V. infusions

- prevent hypothermia, coagulopathy, arrhythmias

Blood Component Therapy
- Fresh Frozen Plasma

  - INR > 1.5 - 2u FFP

- INR 2-2.5 - 4u FFP

- INR > 2.5 - 6u FFP

■ Cryoprecipitate (1u/ 10Kg)

- Fibrinogen < 100 mg/dl – 10u cryo

- Fibrinogen < 50 mg/dl – 20u cryo

■ Platelets

- Platelet. count. < 100,000 – 1u plateletpheresis

- Platelet. count. < 50,000 – 2u plateletpheresis

Blood Comp	Contents	Volume (ml)
Packed RBCs	RBC, Plasma	300
Platelets	Platelets, Plasma	250

FFP	Fibrinogen, antithrombin III, clotting factors, plasma	250
Cryoprecipitate	Fibrinogen, Von Willebrand F, Factor V111, X111, Fibronectin	40

- Maintain systolic BP>90 mmHg

- Maintain urine output > 0.5 ml per kg per hour

- Hct > 21%

- Platelets > 50,000/ul

- Fibrinogen > 100 mg/dl

- PT/PTT < 1.5 times control

- Repeat labs as needed – every 30 minutes

Recombinant factor VIIa (rFVIIa)

1. rFVIIa will not replace ligatures in controlling bleeding from damaged or torn vessels.

2. To be effective there must be adequate circulation delivering platelets and fibrinogen to the site of bleeding.

3. *You should make your best efforts to correct acidosis and hypothermia.*

Causes of Failure of conservative approach

- Uterine rupture
- Placenta accreta

Risk of delaying radical treatment

- Placenta accreta is a frequent cause of failure of conservative Treatments

- Hysterectomy may be a life-saving procedure in

Treatment of the cause

a. Repair

b. Uterine Tamponade (78%)

c. B-Lynch Suture (81%)

d. Arterial Ligation

e. Radiological Arterial Embolization

f. Hysterectomy (12%)

Management of Postoperative bleeding,

- **Surgery** may be done in the same area to pinpoint where the blood is coming from.

- How postoperative bleeding is treated?

- **A blood transfusion**

- **Blood components** may be given during a transfusion to help stop the bleeding.

- Blood components are the parts of blood that help it to clot. Examples are clotting factors, platelets, and plasma.

Types *of blood transfusion*

Donor transfusion.

Side effects of blood transfusion

Allergic reaction

- This type of reaction is usually treated with antihistamines.

- More serious allergic reaction causes difficulty breathing, low blood pressure and nausea.

- Allergic reactions: Diphenhydramine is usually effective for relieving pruritus that is associated with hives or a rash. The route (oral or intravenous) and the dose (25-100 mg) depend on the severity of the reaction and the weight of the patient.

Anaphylactic reactions

- A subcutaneous injection of epinephrine (0.3-0.5 mL of a 1:1000 aqueous solution) is standard treatment.
- If the patient is sufficiently hypotensive to raise the question of the efficacy of the subcutaneous route, epinephrine (0.5 mL of a 1:10,000 aqueous solution) may be administered intravenously.
- Theoretical considerations cause most clinicians to include an infusion of hydrocortisone or prednisolone if an immediate response to epinephrine does not occur

Fever

- It is a febrile transfusion reaction.
- Stop the transfusion to do further tests before deciding whether to continue.
- A febrile reaction can also occur shortly after the transfusion.
- Fever may be accompanied by chills and shaking.

- Febrile, non hemolytic reactions: Usually, fever resolves in 15-30 minutes without specific treatment. If fever causes discomfort, oral acetaminophen (325-500 mg) may be administered. Avoid aspirin because of its prolonged adverse effect on platelet function

Haemolytic reaction

- The transfused red blood cells because the donor blood type is not a good match.

- In response, the immune system attacks the transfused red blood cells, which are viewed as foreign.

- These destroyed cells release a substance into the blood that harms kidneys.

- This usually occurs during or right after a transfusion. Signs and symptoms include fever, nausea, chills, lower back or chest pain, and dark urine

- Acute hemolytic reactions (antibody mediated)
  - Immediately discontinue the transfusion while maintaining venous access for emergency management.
  - Anticipate hypotension, renal failure, and DIC.

- Prophylactic measures to reduce the risk of renal failure may include low-dose dopamine (1-5 mcg/kg/min), vigorous hydration with crystalloid solutions (3000 mL/m^2/24 h), and osmotic diuresis with 20% mannitol (100 mL/m^2/bolus, followed by 30 mL/m^2/h for 12 h).
- If DIC is documented and bleeding requires treatment, transfusions of frozen plasma, pooled cryoprecipitates for fibrinogen, and/or platelet concentrates may be indicated.

Acute hemolytic reactions (non antibody mediated)

- The transfusion of serologically compatible, although damaged, RBCs usually does not require rigorous management.
- Diuresis induced by an infusion of 500 mL of 0.9% sodium chloride per hour, or as tolerated by the patient, until the intense red color of hemoglobinuria ceases is usually adequate treatment.

Delayed hemolytic reaction

This type of reaction is similar to an acute immune hemolytic reaction, but it occurs much more slowly. Your body gradually attacks the donor red blood cells. It could take one to four weeks to notice a decrease in red blood cell levels.

Lung injury

- Transfusion-related acute lung injury (TRALI) is thought to occur due to antibodies or other biologic substances in the blood components.

- With TRALI, the lungs become damaged, making it difficult to breathe. Usually, TRALI occurs within one to six hours of the transfusion. People usually recover, especially when treated quickly.

- Most people who die after TRALI were very sick before the transfusion.

Management of TRALI

- Immediately discontinue the transfusion while preserving venous access.
- Patients with mild episodes should respond to oxygen administered by nasal catheter or mask.

- If shortness of breath persists after oxygen administration, transfer the patient to an intensive care setting where mechanical ventilation can be administered

- In the absence of signs of acute volume overload or cardiogenic pulmonary edema, diuretics are not indicated.
- No evidence exists that corticosteroids or antihistamines are beneficial.
- Treat complications with specific supportive measures.

Circulatory (volume) overload

- Move the patient to a sitting position, and administer oxygen to facilitate breathing.
- Discontinuing the transfusion and removing the excessive fluid.
- The unit of blood component being transfused may be lowered to reverse the flow and to decrease intravascular volume by a controlled phlebotomy.

Blood borne infections

- Blood banks screen donors for risk factors and test donated blood to reduce the risk of transfusion-related infections.

- Infections related to blood transfusion still rarely may occur. It can take weeks or months after a blood transfusion to determine that you've been infected with a virus, bacterium or parasite.

The National Institutes of Health offers the following estimates for the risk of a blood donation carrying an infectious disease:

- HIV — 1 in 2 million donations, which is lower than the risk of being killed by lightning

- Hepatitis B — 1 in 205,000 donations

- Hepatitis C — 1 in 2 million donations

Iron overload

If you receive multiple blood transfusions, you may end up with too much iron in your blood. Iron overload (hemochromatosis) can damage parts of your body, including the liver and the heart. You may receive iron chelation therapy, which uses medication to remove excess iron.

Graft-versus-host disease

Transfusion-associated graft-versus-host disease is a very rare condition in which transfused white blood cells attack the recipient's bone marrow. This disease is usually fatal. It is more likely to affect people with severely weakened immune systems, such as those being treated for leukemia or lymphoma. Signs and symptoms include fever, rash, diarrhea and abnormal liver function test results. Irradiating the blood before transfusing it reduces the risk.

Bacterial contamination (sepsis)

- Immediately discontinue the transfusion, including all tubing, filters, and administration sets, and save the transfusion materials for cultures, while preserving venous access.
- After appropriate blood cultures have been obtained, initiate treatment with intravenous broad-spectrum antibiotics.
- If a microbiologic stain or a culture of the contents of the transfused product identifies an organism, the initial broad-spectrum antibacterial approach may be modified accordingly.

Consultation

- Medical director of the hospital's blood bank or a designee (e.g., a clinical pathology resident, transfusion medicine fellow).
- the blood bank consultant may arrange for microbiologic stains and cultures of the residual contents of the blood product container,

Clerical checks for patient and product identification in the laboratory, repeat compatibility testing using a freshly collected blood sample from the recipient, or other pertinent diagnostic studies.

- The diagnosis of an acute hemolytic transfusion reaction should trigger consultation with a nephrologist to ensure optimal prophylactic measures to prevent renal damage.
- A hematology consultation is appropriate if a hemolytic transfusion reaction or bacterial contamination precipitated DIC.
- A clinical diagnosis of bacterial contamination of a transfused blood product should trigger an infectious diseases consultation.

Autologous blood transfusion.

- Blood collection begins three to five weeks before elective surgery, depending on the number of units required, usually 2-4 units (about 1-2 litres).

- The last donation takes place at least 48-72 hours before surgery to allow for re-equilibration of the blood volume

Advantages of Autologous blood transfusion

1. Predeposit autologous transfusion virtually eliminates the risks of viral transmission and immunologically mediated hemolytic, febrile, or allergic reactions.

2. These adverse effects range in frequency y from 1 in 1 000 000 (HIV) to as high as 5% (febrile reactions). In addition, it may decrease the risk of postoperative infection and recurrence of cancer because immunomodulation as a result of transfusion is avoided.

3. Immunomodulation refers to decreases in cellular immune function that have been documented after allogeneic, but not autologous, transfusions.[7]

Disadvantages

1. Up to half of the blood that is collected may be discarded because the amount drawn off needs to exceed the median routinely needed to avoid additional allogeneic transfusions.

2. Leftover blood can rarely be used for other patients because most autologous donors do not meet the stringent health requirements for allogeneic blood donation.

3. This wastage of blood and the costs of administering autologous programs result in collection costs that are higher than those for allogeneic transfusion.

4. Volume overload, bacterial contamination, and ABO hemolytic reactions to the transfusion resulting from administrative or clerical errors are further risks.

5. Timing of autologous transfusion

   Pre-operative donation: donating of the blood before surgery. The blood bank draws your blood and stores it until you need it during or after surgery.

   - This option is only for non-emergency (elective) surgery.

Intra-operative autologous transfusion:

   - Recycling of the blood during surgery. Blood lost during surgery is filtered, and put back into your body during surgery.

   - This can be done in emergency and elective surgeries.

- Post-operative autologous transfusion: recycling your blood after surgery. Blood lost after surgery is collected, filtered and returned to your body.

Hem dilution:

- Restricted to patients in whom substantial blood loss is predicted (>1 liter or 20% of blood volume).

- Whole blood (1.0-1.5 liters) is removed, and simultaneously intravascular volume is replaced with crystalloid or colloid, or both, to maintain blood volume.

- The anticoagulated blood is then reinfused in the operating theatre during or shortly after surgical blood loss has stopped.

Disadvantages

1. The circulating red cell mass is lowered appreciably and acutely.

2. If colloid is used for volume replacement the risk of allergic reactions or hemostatic abnormalities increases.

3. expense of, and inconvenience to, the anesthetist who performs the procedure

<u>Apheresis</u>: donating platelets and plasma.

Before surgery, the platelets and plasma, which help stop bleeding, are withdrawn, filtered and returned to the patient.

- **Antifibrinolytic medicines** may slow or stop the bleeding.

- **Surgery** may be done to fix the blood vessel or area that is bleeding

- **Pulmonary Embolism**

  1. Pulmonary embolism,
  2. Amniotic fluid embolism
  3. Air embolism

Pulmonary embolism

40% of asymptomatic patients with DVT have radio graphically documented pulmonary embolism

• DVT of pelvic venous system is often an asymptomatic condition until clinical pulmonary embolism develops

Risk factors

Many have been identified in medical patients resulting in an increase in VTE rates and mortality.

- Higher age
- Cancer
- Immobilization

- Infectious disease
- a history of VTE
- Inherited thrombophilia is another established risk factor of VTE.

- those admitted to an Intensive Care Unit (ICU) represent a high risk population for VTE [10-13] with a higher prevalence of the aforementioned risk factors

Relative risk factors

- Smoker
- Diabetes mellitus
- Renal insufficiency
- high APACHE-II-Score

Laboratory risks

- Laboratory results D-dimere (increased vs. normal)
- CRP (increased vs. normal)
- Leukocytes (increased vs. normal)
- Fibrinogen (increased vs. normal)
- PTT (increased vs. normal)
- Erythrocytes (increased vs. normal)
- Creatinine (increased vs. normal)

- Thrombocytes (increased vs. normal)
- Quick (decreased vs. normal)

• Untreated pulmonary embolism mortality is up to 30%. Treated mortality is 3%

(Moser et al, 1994; Cunningham et al, 1997; Toglia & Weg, 1996)

Thromboprophylaxis

- Thromboprophylaxis is important in   critically ill patients because of their high risk of venous thromboembolism
- The Joint Commission now specifies thromboprophylaxis as a key quality measure for hospitalized patients

Types of Thromboprophylaxis

Pharmacologic prophylaxis

Pharmacologic prophylaxis (UFH, LMWH, warfarin, danaparoid, other agents),

Mechanical prophylaxis

- Mechanical prophylaxis (antiembolic stockings, pneumatic compression devices)
- therapeutic anticoagulation
- antiplatelet treatments
- use of inferior vena cava filters were captured daily,

Follow up of Thromboprophylaxis

- laboratory values (for example, platelet count)

- outcomes (for example, bleeding)

- confirmatory tests (for all venous thromboembolism events)

- Process of care variables (for example, mobility).

- Thromboprophylaxis was administered using preprinted orders or computerized physician order entry.

Clinical manifestations of pulmonary embolism

Hypotension or cardiogenic shock, due to acute cor pulmonale (ACP)

Pulmonary embolism severity index

1. Age >80 years

2. History of cancer

3. History of heart failure or chronic lung disease

4. Pulse rate ≥110 bpm

5. Systolic blood pressure <100 mmHg

6. Oxygen saturation <90 % on room air

7. Right ventricular dysfunction (RVD) assessed by echocardiography or spiral computed tomography angiography

8. biomarkers including brain natriuretic peptide (BNP), N-terminal pro-BNP (NT-proBNP) and troponin

9. cardiogenic shock

10. Recurrent PE in patients with normal blood pressure.

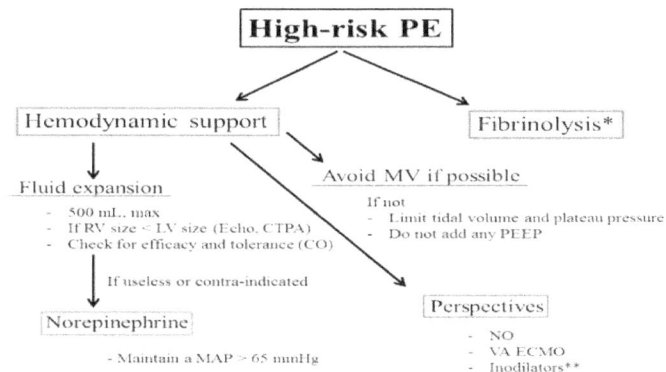

Clinical picture of pulmonary embolism

Acute hypotension

Cardiac arrest

Acute hypoxia

Cyanosis

Respiratory arrest

Coagulopathy

Defined as laboratory evidence of intravascular consumption or fibrinolysis or sever clinical hemorrhage in absence of

Onset during dilation and evacuation, labor cesarean section delivery, or within 30 minute post-partum

Amniotic Fluid Embolism (*Anaphylactoid syndrome of pregnancy*)

Frequency- 1/15,000 - 1/20,000 Pregnancies

- unpredictable
- unpreventable and an untreatable
- Catastrophic Consequences
- Multisystem Collapse
- Mortality Quoted as High as 80%
- (Probably Lower Now)

  <u>Theoretical causes</u>

1) Uterine Hyper stimulation AFE registry suggests that hyper stimulation is EFFECT rather than cause of AFE
2) Oxytocin use- NOT RELATED
3) Drug Allergy and/or Atopy- RELATED, with 41% of patients in AFE registry with allergies
4) Normal labor

The classic clinical presentation of the syndrome has been described by five signs that often occur in the following sequence:

   a. Respiratory distress
   b. Cyanosis
   c. Cardiovascular collapse *cardiogenic shock*
   d. Hemorrhage
   e. Seizure & Coma.

- The presence of squamous cells in the pulmonary arterial blood obtained from a Swan-Ganz catheter once considered pathognomonic for AFE is neither sensitive nor specific

- The monoclonal antibody TKAH-2 may eventually prove more useful in the rapid diagnosis of AFE

Diagnosis of Pulmonary Embolism

- D-dimer (0-300 ng/ml as normal)
- Chest X-ray
- ECG
- Arterial blood gas
- Ventilation-perfusion scintography
- Angiography
- Thoracic enhanced CT (64 slices)
- Extremity Doppler

Recent guidelines of the European Society of Cardiology recommended the following support:

(1) Use volume expansion with caution,

(2 use norepinephrine infusion to improve RV function if necessary when blood pressure is low,

(3) ventilate patients, when required, with a low tidal volume and plateau pressure.

Vena cava filter

The only indication for filter placement recommended by all guidelines is the contraindication to anticoagulant treatment in patients with PE or proximal DVT

Risk factors for Venous Air Embolism

Mortality of VAE ranges from 48 to 80%.

High risk surgeries for VAE

- o Sitting position and posterior fossa neurosurgeries, cesarean section,
- o laparoscopic
- o orthopedic
- o Surgeries invasive procedures
- o Pulmonary overpressure syndrome
- o Decompression syndrome.
- o Operative site 5 cm above the heart
- o Creation of pressure gradient which will facilitate entry of air into the circulation
- o orogenital sex during pregnancy

- Rapid ascent in scuba (self contained underwater breathing apparatus) divers and barotrauma or chest trauma.
- Large bolus of air can lead to right ventricular air lock and immediate fatality.
- In up to 35% patient, the foramen ovale is patent which can cause paradoxical arterial air embolism
- bronchogenic cyst or cystic air filled lesion in the lung.

Diagnosis of VAE

- High index of clinical suspicion
- The transesophgeal echocardiography to detect smallest amount of air in the circulation

The cardiac manifestations

- chest pain,

- Brady arrhythmias

- tachyarrhythmia's,

- Increased filling pressure due to right sided heart failure and in late stage typical mill-wheel murmur.

o   Electrocardiogram may show s-t segment changes or right ventricular strain pattern.

The pulmonary changes

o   dyspnoea,

o   tachypnoea

o   'gasp' reflex as a result of acute hypoxaemia or even pulmonary edema.

o   Patient may have reduced lung compliance, increased dead space and acute shunting leading to hypoxaemia and hypercarbia

Causes of Neurological manifestations

- first the cardiovascular collapse causing reduced cardiac output leading to cerebral hypo-perfusion, secondly
- Direct paradoxical cerebral embolism may occur through patent foramen ovale.

Treatment of VAE

Prevent further entrainment of air and reduce the volume of air entrained

- **prevention of VAE**

- proper positioning during surgery,
- optimal hydration,
- avoiding use of nitrous oxide,
- meticulous care during insertion, removal of central venous catheter
- proper guidance,
- Training of scuba divers.

Treatment

- Administration of 100% oxygen will maximize the patient's oxygenation as well as reduces embolus volume by eliminating nitrogen

- By maintaining the systemic arterial pressure with optimal fluid status

- inotropic support to the heart will help by keeping the patient stable partial left lateral decubitus position

- Trendelenburg's position as a favourable placement to optimize hemodynamic is now controversial.

- Aspiration of air from right atrium is possibly best treatment to improve the haemodynamic parameters immediately and this can be done, with use of Bunegin-Albin multiorifice catheter up to 60% success rate.

- Rapid cardiopulmonary resuscitation with chest compression demonstrated to be effective in massive VAE which result in cardiac standstill.

- Hyperbaric oxygen therapy in the cases of VAE is beneficial as it causes compression of existing air bubbles, by establishing a high diffusion gradient to speed dissolution of bubbles and by improving oxygenation in the ischemic tissues.

- The early compression therapy has better results, as per Boyle's law,

- Anticoagulation therapy with heparin in patients with air embolism decreases the severity of the disease, if treated with heparin before air embolization

- As steroids do not have any effect on cytotoxic brain edema which occurs in the patients with air emboilsm, the use of steroid is controversial

- Prophylactic lidocain is effective in reducing the gas embolism effect on brain, it deceases brain edema in experimental animals. Various case reports suggesting that the lignocain has beneficial effect in patient with decompression syndrome.

- **LABS: CBC, ABG, PT, PTT, fibrinogen, FDP.**

- **Cardiac output with crystalloids.**

- **After correction of hypotension, restrict fluid therapy to maintenance levels since ARDS follows in up to 40% to 70% of cases.**

- **Dopamine infusion if patient remains hypotensive (myocardial support).**

- **vasopressor therapy such as ephedrine with success (reduced systemic vascular resistance)**

Septic Shock

Sepsis is a potentially life-threatening medical condition that's associated with an infection

- **bacterial infections**,
- **fungal infections**,
- Other causes of infection or agents that may cause SIRS.
- organ location or implanted device (for example, skin, lung **pneumonia**
- gastrointestinal tract [bacterial penetration
- ruptured intestine from **trauma**
- surgical site, intravenous catheter
- The infecting agents or their toxins (or both)

Stages of sepsis

The first stage

It is the least severe and usually has symptoms of fever and an increased heart rate.

The second stage is more severe and is characterized by symptoms of difficulty breathing and possible organ malfunctions,

The third is the most severe stage (septic shock) with life-threatening low blood pressure

Clinical picture of sepsis

- altered mental status,
- increased respiratory rate,
- Low blood pressure.
- Pulse
- Blood Pressure
- Temperature
- Respiratory rate

Risk factors for sepsis

The following groups are at increased risk for sepsis:

- The very young and the elderly are at greatest risk

- People who are very ill due to an infectious agent

- People in an intensive-care unit

- People with weakened or compromised immune systems

- People with devices such as IV catheters, breathing tubes, or other devices

- People with extensive burns

- People with severe trauma

Causes of septicemia

- **MRSA** sepsis: sepsis caused by methicillin-resistant *Staphylococcus aureus* bacteria

- **VRE** sepsis: sepsis caused by **vancomycin-**resistant *Enterococcus* species of bacteria

- Urosepsis: sepsis originating from a **urinary tract infection (UTI)**

- **Wound** sepsis: sepsis originating from an infection of a wound

- Neonatal sepsis or septicemia: sepsis seen in newborns, usually in the first four weeks after birth; sepsis neonatorum means the same as neonatal sepsis

- Septic abortion: an abortion due to infection with sepsis in the mother

Treatment

- Antibiotics within the **'Golden Hour'**

    - Time to administration is a predictor of mortality. From time of diagnosis each hour's delay in administration of antibiotics

- increases the chance of death by 8%.(Kumar et al. Crit Care Med. 2006,34;1589-1596)

- Initially broad spectrum then narrowed as results from microbiology become available

- **Strong indicator of multi-organ failure**

- > 1mmol/L occurs in sepsis

- > 4mmol/L establishes severe sepsis

  Postnatal - there may be a transient rise in lactate BUT do not dismiss if signs of infection or the rise is sustained

- IV fluid bolus to support the circulation

- Appropriate on going monitoring – Pulse, Blood Pressure, Urine output.

- If the response is not sustained then consider inotropes and invasive monitoring

Septicaemia

Recommendations

- **Early advice** from an **infectious diseases** physician or **microbiologist** should be shared in the the choice of antibiotic may need to be adjusted to widen the spectrum of organisms being covered and/or in light of the suspected source of infection.

- Clinicians should not only **document an action plan** in the case record but **initiate the actions** required such as the administration of antibiotics and the commencement of fluids.

- It is recommended that **education on the recognition and treatment of sepsis** is integrated into the annual training already taking place for all staff caring for pregnant women, especially for those practicing in 'low risk' settings.

- Correct and repeated risk assessments.

- Inappropriate ward settings for pregnant women

    Recommendation

- All **consultant led delivery suites** must have access to a place **appropriately equipped and staffed by teams of senior obstetricians, anaesthetists and midwives, skilled in looking after seriously ill women** especially those with sepsis. Plans should be in place for provision of critical care on delivery units if this is the most appropriate setting for a woman with sepsis to receive care.

- **Act quickly with therapeutics**

- **Measure & Monitor all vital signs**

- **Obtain senior expert advice**

- Early in sepsis there is an increase in inflammatory mediators

- Mid- to late sepsis consistent with immunosuppression

  - loss of hypersensitivity

  - inability to clear infection

  - predisposition to nosocomial infections

  - Non-responsiveness to antigen

  - T cells fail to proliferate and secrete cytokines in response to antigen

- Death of immune cells

  - Apoptosis (suicide or programmed cell death)

  - Decrease in B cells, CD4 T cells and follicular dendritic cells

- The normal stress response is activation of anti-inflammatory mechanisms which predominate in sites outside of the affected systems

  - Not the previously believed uncontrolled hyperinflammatory response

- Survival among patients correlates with recovery of inflammatory responses

- Shock: When the <u>functional</u> intravascular blood volume is below that of the capacity of the body's vascular bed

  - Hypovolemic

  - Hemorrhagic

  - Cardiogenic (pump failure)

  - Neurogenic (loss of sympathetic control of <u>resistance vessels)</u>

Systemic Inflammatory Response Syndrome (SIRS)

  - Inflammatory process that can be generated by infection or by non-infectious causes (burns, trauma)

  - **Non-pregnant**: 2 or more of the following

    - Temperature >38 C or <36 C

    - HR > 90 beats/min

    - RR >20 breaths/min

    - WBC > 12,000/mm^3, < 4,000/mm^3

- Sepsis : the systemic inflammatory response syndrome that occurs during infection (Society Critical Care Medicine 2001 consensus statement)

- Septic shock: vascular collapse secondary to an infectious process

    - Usually components of hypovolemic and cardiogenic shock

- Septic shock: 0.002-0.01% of all deliveries

- 0.3-0.6% of all septic patients are pregnant

- Has increased over the last decade

    - Older maternal age at delivery

        - Obesity, diabetes, placental abruption and placenta accreta

        - ART and multi-fetal gestation

    - Obesity

        - DM, Cesarean, cardiopulmonary complications

Bacterial Infections in Obstetrics

- Postpartum endometritis

-   – Cesarean delivery   15-87 %

-   – Vaginal delivery   1-4 %

- Lower tract UTI   1-4 %

- Septic abortion   1-2 %

- Pyelonephritis   1-2 %

- Chorioamnionitis   0.5 - 1 %

- Necrotizing fasciitis   < 1 %

- Toxic shock syndrome   < 1

- **Common Bacterial Isolates from OB Patients with Septic Shock**

- *Escherichia coli*

- Group B streptococci

- *Bacteroides* spp.

- *Peptostreptococcus*

- *Peptococcus* spp.

- *Clostridium perfringens*

- Group A streptoco

Entercoccus spp.

    Staphylococcus aureus

Listeria monocytogenes

Klebsiella pneumoniae

Pseudomonas aeruginosa

Enterbacter spp.

Proteus spp.

Clinical Manifestations

- Early stages
    - RECOGNITION KEY TO SUCCESSFUL TREATMENT
    - Shaking chills, fever (most common in pregnancy), tachycardia, flushing
    - Warm extremities, nausea, vomiting, diarrhea
    - slight changes in mental status
    - May be difficult to diagnose early in pregnant women, particularly in labor
- Laboratory findings
    - mild leukopenia or leukocytosis, hyperglycemia
    - early DIC : thrombocytopenia, decreased fibrinogen, increased PTT and PT
    - transient respiratory alkalosis with increasing metabolic acidosis
        - Increased serum lactate
        - Low arterial pH
        - Increased base deficit
- Laboratory findings

- mild leukopenia or leukocytosis, hyperglycemia
- early DIC : thrombocytopenia, decreased fibrinogen, increased PTT and PT
- transient respiratory alkalosis with increasing metabolic acidosis
    - Increased serum lactate
    - Low arterial pH
    - Increased base deficit

Multiple Organ Effects with Sepsis and Shock

- CNS Effects : Confusion, coma, fever
- Cardiovascular: Hypotension, increased CO, myocardial depression tachyarrhythmia
- Pulmonary: Hypoxemia, diffuse infiltrates
- Renal: Hypoperfusion, acute tubular necrosis
- Hematologic: Thrombocytopenia, leukocytosis, consumptive coagulopathy

Laboratory Evaluation

- Complete blood count
    - differential and platelets
- Coagulation profile
    - PT,PTT, Fibrinogen

- Electrolytes, glucose

- Creatinine

- Urinalysis and culture

- Blood culture and gram stain

- Cultures of infected sites

- Chest X-ray

  Causes of death

- CT, ultrasound, MRI to localize infectious etiology

- Myocardial depression : Cardiac output usually maintained due to tachycardia and cardiac dilitation

- ARDS : death rare from hypoxemia or hypercarbia

- Renal failure : dialysis will prevent death

- Liver dysfunction : hepatic encephalopathy rare

Management of septic shock
- Volume resuscitation

  – Aggressive therapy will optimize afterload, preload and cardiac contractility

  – Normalize mixed venous oxygen saturation, lactate concentrations and pH

- Blood products, colloid, crystalloid

- Oxygenation/Ventilation

  - Mechanical ventilation usually required

  - ARDS : hypoxemia, diffuse infiltrates and decreased pulmonary compliance

  - Keep at or above 96% if possible during pregnancy

  - Blood transfusion can increase O_2 content : keep Hgb ~ 10 g/dl

- Inotropic agents

  - Dopamine hydrochloride (a-adrenergic and b-adrenergic effects)

  - Dobutamine

  - Norepinephrine – now considered first line therapy

    - Increases mean arterial pressure

    - Can reduce uterine artery blood flow

- Empiric antibiotic therapy

  - Find the underlying etiology of the sepsis

  - Start broad spectrum antibiotics immediately after drawing cultures

- Penicillin (if *Staphylococcus aureus* suspected, consider Vancomycin) or derivative PLUS aminoglycoside PLUS Clindamycin
  - Alter regimen as culture and sensitivity results available
- Surgical drainage or removal of infected tissues
  - uterine evacuation, hysterectomy, abscess drainage, etc depending on the etiology
- Corticosteroids: high doses do not increase survival. Physiologic doses may be beneficial in extremely ill patients (relative adrenal insufficiency)
- Activated Protein C
  - First anti-inflammatory agent effective in the treatment of septic shock (NEJM 2001)
  - Inactivates Factors Va and VIIIa, preventing thrombin generation
  - 3.5% risk of serious hemorrhage
  - However, U.S. FDA, based on the PROWESS-SHOCK clinical trial, issued a statement in 2011 that it should not be started in new patients with sepsis because it failed to show a survival benefit

- Activated Protein C

    - First anti-inflammatory agent effective in the treatment of septic shock (NEJM 2001)

    - Inactivates Factors Va and VIIIa, preventing thrombin generation

    - 3.5% risk of serious hemorrhage

- Controlling chronic disease

- Antimicrobial prophylaxis

    - Repeat if case > 4 hours

    - Increase dose in obese patients

- A standardized approach should be formulated for pregnant women with suspected sepsis

    - Early diagnosis procedures

    - Management protocol to include both maternal and fetal evaluation and treatment

Anesthesia and septic shock

Preoperative measures for septic shock patien

The timely administration of appropriate i.v. antimicrobial therapy is a crucial step in the care of patients with severe sepsis who may require surgery to control the source of sepsis.

Preoperative resuscitation,

Optimizing major organ perfusion, is based on judicious use of fluids, vasopressors, and inotropes.

Intraoperative anesthesia management

- Requires careful induction and maintenance of anesthesia,
- optimizing intravascular volume status,
- avoidance of lung injury during mechanical ventilation,
- monitoring
- arterial blood gases,
- lactate concentration,
- hematological
- renal indices,
- Electrolyte levels.
- Most anesthetic induction agents cause blood pressure decline,
- It may be useful to use drugs, such as ketamine or etomidate, which carry less cardiovascular instability effects than propofol, thiopental and midazolam.
- However, if blood pressure is unstable, despite these efforts, vasopressors and inotropic agents must be administered to maintain adequate perfusion of organs and cellular oxygen uptake.

- Anesthesiologist should evaluate the myocardial performance and hemodynamic monitoring for preload estimation of the patient by inserting a CVP catheter and evaluating the volume status.
- However, because it is difficult to accurately evaluate the intravascular volume only by CVP measurements, the additional use of transthoracic echocardiography, which the ventricular filling, ventricular function can be evaluated.
- An arterial catheter is rapidly placed in order to assess the blood pressure in septic shock patients.

Postoperative care

- Management of the severe sepsis syndrome patient in the intensive care unit.
- already requiring multiple supports, and require experienced and skilful decision-making to optimize their chances of a favourable outcome.

Anaphylaxis and anesthesia

- The incidence of anaphylaxis during anesthesia ranges from 1 in 4000 to 1 in 25,000.
- Anaphylaxis generally occurs on re-exposure to a specific antigen and requires the release of proinflammatory mediators, but it can also occur on first exposure, because there is cross-reactivity among many commercial products and drugs.

immune-mediated allergic reactions are classified

Type I immunoglobulin (Ig)E-mediated hypersensitivity reaction

involving mast cells and basophils, contact dermatitis is a Type IV T-lymphocyte cell-mediated delayed-type hypersensitivity reaction.

Type II reactions

IgG, IgM, and complement mediate cytotoxicity

Type III reactions

- immune-complex formation and deposition leads to tissue damage
- Anaphylactic reactions occur through a direct nonimmune-mediated release of mediators from mast cells and/or basophils or result from direct complement activation.

- Activation of tyrosine kinases and calcium influx in mast cells and basophils result in rapid release of granule associated preformed mediators such as histamine, tryptase, carboxypeptidase A3, chymase, and proteoglycans.

- activation of phospholipase A2, COXs, and lipoxygenases leads to production of arachidonic acid metabolites

- Prostaglandins and leukotrienes and synthesis of the platelet-activating factor.

- Cytokines and chemokines are synthesized and released, including IL-6, the newly recognized IL-33 and TNF-a, which is both a late-phase mediator and a preformed mediator.

- The opening of the endothelial barrier through endothelial Gq/G11-mediated signaling has been identified.

Intraoperative causes of anaphylaxix

Drugs,

- Colloids , Dextran and hydroxyethyl starch (HES), large-molecularweight polysaccharides, may be used as a nonblood, highoncotic fluid replacement during surgery

- Exposed to natural latex rubber. Latex allergy should also be considered when gynaecological procedures are performed. Particles from obstetricians' gloves, which accumulate in the uterus during obstetrical manoeuvres, could suddenly be released into the systemic blood flow following oxytocin injection.

- Anesthetic drugs, neuromuscular blocking agents (muscle relaxants), which are responsible for 60% to 70% of episodes of anaphylaxis occurring during this period. Neuromuscular blocking agents can induce two types of reactions. One is driven by an immunological mechanism and is IgE-dependent with the quaternary ammonium (NH4 +) structures as main antigenic epitope. while the second one, particularly described with benzylisoquinolinium-type NMBA such as mivacurium, atracurium, and d-tubocurarine, results from nonspecific stimulation of mast cells Cross-reactivity between NMBA is said to be common

   Antibiotics, Anaphylactic reactions to antibiotics have also been reported following removal of tourniquet during orthopaedic surgery. Penicillin, cephalosporins, and other-lactam antibiotics

Sulfonamide allergy

Vancomycin is a glycopeptide antibiotic selectively used for treatment of resistant organisms and for use in individuals with penicillin allergy.

Induction drugs

Barbiturates, especially thiopental

- **Propofol** may directly stimulate histamine release, and this effect may be greater when administered with muscle relaxants.

- **Diazepam** is more likely than midazolam to cause an anaphylactic reaction because of the propylene glycol solvent that replaced Cremophor EL.

- Morphine is a tertiary amine that causes nonimmunological histamine release, and meperidine causes nonimmunological histamine release more often than any other opioid. There are reported cases of IgE-mediated reactions to these opioids.

- Agents include: Acetylcholine, choline, morphine, neostigmine, and pentolinium. Cross-inhibition suggests that previous exposure to these nonanesthetic drugs may sensitize individuals to muscle-relaxing agents, resulting in reactions among patients without prior anesthesia.

- *Local anesthetic agents* readily induce cell-mediated immunologic reactions when applied topically to the skin, but humoral immune responses are rare.

- Povidone-iodine

Povidone-iodine (betadine) is the most common topical antiseptic solution use. Allergic contact dermatitis, a Type IV cell-mediated hypersensitivity reaction,

- implanted antimicrobial surgical mesh, and insertion of chlorhexidine-coated central venous catheters Other

Diagnosis of intraoperative anaphylaxis

- Diagnosis of anaphylaxis during anesthesia is not easy. It can be difficult as different drugs can provoke mixed allergic and nonallergic reactions with different pathological mechanisms
- Past history of the patient of allergy to certain drugs and antibiotics, or injection of dye during diagnostic procedures, and history of bronchial asthma ,atopic dermatits
- **By timing after exposure to certain drugs**
  The timing in relation to drug administration is important, and gives a clue to the aetiology.

minutes of induction

Intravenous anesthetics, Intravenous opiate, and Intravenous antibiotic

intraoperatively

IV NSAIDs, opiods, antibiotics.

At end of surgery or during recovery

Latex allergy, rectal NSAID and IV opioids are the cause

Investigations :

- None of the available diagnostic tests demonstrates absolute accuracy.
- False-positive test results may merely cause an inconvenience (unnecessary avoidance of a safe drug), whereas false-negative or equivocal results may be extremely dangerous and severely undermine correct secondary prevention.
- Series of investigations performed both immediately and days to weeks later.
- **Biological investigations**
  - mediator release assays at the time of the reaction , quantification of specific IgE, immediately or 6 weeks later
  - skin tests

- other biological assays such as histamine release tests or basophil activation assays
- Early tests are essentially designed to determine whether or not an immunological mechanism is involved.

- Delayed skin tests attempt to identify the responsible drug.

1. **<u>Differential diagnosis of anaphylaxis during anesthesia</u>**
2. Drug overdose
3. interactions Cardiac/vascular drug effects
4. Asthma
5. Arrhythmia
6. Myocardial infarction
7. Pericardial tamponade
8. Pulmonary edema
9. Pulmonary embolism
10. Tension pneumothorax
11. Hemorrhagic shock
12. Venous embolism
13. Sepsis
14. C1-esterase inhibitor deficiency

15. Mastocytosis

16. **Malignant hyperthermia** (succinylcholine) Myotonias and masseter spasm (succinylcholine) Hyperkaliemia (succinylcholine)

Grade of severity for quantification of immediate hypersensitivity reactions.

a. **Generalized cutaneous signs :**

Erythema, urticaria, with or without angioedema

b. **Moderate multiorgan involvement** with cutaneous signs, hypotension and tachycardia, bronchial hyperreactivity : cough, difficulty to inflate

c. **Severe life-threatening** s multiorgan involvement: collapse, tachycardia or bradycardia, arrhythmias, bronchospasm. Cutaneous signs may be present or occur only after the arterial blood pressure recovers

d. **Cardiac and/or respiratory arrest**

Clinical manifestation,

Cardiovascular

- Loss of pulse
- Hypotension
- Arrhythmia
- Ventricular fibrillation

Respiratory

- Difficulty in lung inflation ,
- brochospasm
- Desaturation.
- A decreased $etCO_2$ value is also of valuable diagnostic parameter.

Management of intraoperative anaphylaxis

Management of patient with suspected anaphylaxis during anesthesia

1. Stop administration of all agents likely to have caused the anaphylaxis.

2. Call for help.

3. Maintain airway, give 100% oxygen and lie patient flat with legs elevated.

4. Give epinephrine (adrenaline). This may be given intramuscularly in a dose of 0.5 mg to 1 mg (0.5 to 1 mL of 1:1,000) and may be repeated every 10 min according to the arterial pressure and pulse until improvement occurs. Alternatively, 50 to 100 µg intravenously (0.5 to 1 mL of 1:10,000) over 1 min has been recommended for hypotension with titration of further doses as required.

Never give undiluted epinephrine 1:1000 intravenously. In a patient with cardiovascular collapse, 0.5 to 1 mg (5 to 10 mL of 1:10,000) may be required intravenously in divided doses by titration. This should be given at a rate of 0.1 mg/min stopping when a response has been obtained. Paediatric doses of epinephrine depend on the age of the child.

Intramuscular epinephrine 1:1000 should be administered as follows

>12 years 500 µg IM (0.5 mL)

6-12 years 250 µg IM (0.25 mL)

>6 months-6 years 120 µg IM (0.12 mL)

<6 months 50 µg IM (0.05 mL)

Start rapid intravenous infusion with colloids or crystalloids.

Adult patients may require 2 to 4 L of crystalloid.

Secondary therapy

1. Give antihistamines (chlorpheniramine 10-20 mg by slow intravenous infusion).

2. Give corticosteroids (100 to 500 mg hydrocortisone slowly iv).

3. Bronchodilators may be required for persistent bronchospasm.

cutaneous, percutaneous, mucosal, and parenteral application. Life-threatening reactions with profound hypotension, ventricular fibrillation and cardiac ischemia are generally associated with mucosal or parenteral exposure as might occur during application of urethral gels, implanted antimicrobial surgical mesh, and insertion of chlorhexidine-coated central venous catheters respectively. Severe, potentially life-threatening anaphylaxis from simple cutaneous application such as perioperative skin disinfection and wound cleansing remains anecdotal and probably underestimated

- **Nonsteroidal anti-inflammatory drugs**

Aspirin and NSAIDs are the second most common cause of drug-induced anaphylaxis (after antibiotics).Anaphylactic reactions to NSAIDs are unrelated to other reactions caused by these drugs, such as respiratory reactions and exacerbations of chronic idiopathic urticaria.

Causes of exaggerated manifestation of anaphylaxis under anesthesia

- Exaggerated pharmacological effect, e.g., hypotension during extradural anesthesia or with propofol; bradycardia and hypotension after opiates

- Anaphylaxis to one of the i.v. NMBAs or anesthetic drugs

- Adverse reaction to another administered drug e.g., drug with premedication; antibiotic with induction; analgesic, e.g., NSAID rectally or opiate intraoperative

- Latex rubber allergy

- Reaction to intravenous infusion, for example colloid, blood, plasma

- Allergy to other substance given, e.g., chlorhexidine or a diagnostic dye

- Problem with anesthetic technique, for example intubation

- Autonomic parasympathetic effects, e.g., during laparoscopy, peritoneal traction, arthroscopy, squint surgery, dental surgery

- Blood loss

- Medical (non-allergic) cause, for example septicemia; cardiac; severe asthma, pneumothorax; air embolus

- Malignant hyperthermia

Perioperative Myocardial infarction

- Myocardial infarction was defined as elevated troponin with clinical, ECG, or imaging evidence of myocardial ischemia.

- The 30-day mortality rate was 5-fold higher in patients with postoperative MI (11.6% vs 2.2%) and was similar between those with and without ischemic symptoms.

- Apart from high mortality, increased surgical morbidity (sepsis, wound infection, pneumonia, and deep vein thrombosis) is common, when IPEMI–POMI occur.

-

Preoperative cardiac assessment

- If emergency operation is needed proceed to the operating room

- If the patient underwent coronary vascularization in the past five years and there is no ischemic attack proceed to the operating room

- If the patent has major predictor and managed well proceed to the operating room

- If the patient has intermediate predictor it must be evaluate the functional class of the heart non-invasively .if less than 4 evaluate invasively

- If the patient has any minor clinical predictor evaluate functional class if less than 4 with high risk surgery consider noninvasive testing low and intermediate surgery proceed to surgery If more than 4 proceed to surgery.

Preoperative and intraoperative management

- Patients received a beta-blocker if they had known coronary artery disease or met 2 of the following criteria: older than 65 years, hypertension, total cholesterol level higher than 6.2 mmol/L, smoking history, or diabetes mellitus.

- Atenolol produced a 15% absolute risk reduction in the end points of MI, unstable angina, CHF requiring hospitalization, or death at 6 months and reduced mortality at 6 months and 2 years in noncardiac surgery.

- Similarly, another randomized controlled trial evaluating the cardio protective effects of bisoprolol in high-risk patients undergoing vascular surgery was performed. The study was stopped early because of the dramatic results

Postoperative management

- The Perioperative Ischemia Research Group evaluated the use of continuous echocardiographic monitoring perioperative and found that ischemia occurred most frequently on postoperative days 1 and 2 (ie, 20% preoperative, 25% intraoperative, 55% postoperative).
- Because postoperative ischemia can be more deleterious than ischemia detected at other times, interventions, including the perioperative use of beta-blockers and high-dose narcotic analgesia to reduce postoperative pain, are recommended.

Risk factors of intraoperative myocardial infarction

- vascular surgery
- Clinically significant preoperative myocardial infarction.
- Stress of surgery (increased intraoperative bleeding and aortic, peripheral vascular, and emergency surgery),
- poor preoperative cardiac functional status (congestive heart failure, lower ejection fraction, diagnosis of coronary artery disease),
- Preoperative history of coronary artery bypass grafting are the factors that determine perioperative cardiac morbidity and mortality rates.

Intraoperative Trans esophageal echo cardio- graphy (IOTEE) provides important information in the operation room, which affects surgical and hemodynamic management.

It facilitates the assessment of the surgical results, the modification of the planned surgical intervention and the detection of complication such as intraoperative myocardial infarction. Once intraoperative myocardial ischemia, especially myocardial infarction, occurs, the hemo-dynamics may become unstable and result in a fatal outcome. Accordingly, rapid diagnose-sis of intraoperative myocardial infarction is indispensable in management of such a case. Accurate assessment of responsible coronary lesion by the preoperative coronary angiography to determine the anatomical site of ischemia.

Address for correspondence and reprint requests: Hiroyoshi Nakajima, M.D., Division of Cardiology, Mitsui Memo-rial Hospital, 1 Kandaizumi-cho, Chiyoda-ku, Tokyo 101-8643, Japan. Fax: +81-3-5687-9765; E-mail: nakaji-tky@ umin.ac.jp

Management of intraoperative myocardial infarction

- Close and continuous monitoring of patients at risk of myocardial ischemia during anesthesia is necessary, using optimal ECG lead configurations, but sensitivity of this monitoring is not 100%.
- Subtle ST-segment changes in electrocardiogram are not always appreciated, unless there is a computerized monitor analysis. The majority of perioperative AMIs are non-Q wave and electrocardiographic changes are therefore non-specific.
- Laboratory values of CPK and CPKMB are not reliable, because of co-existing muscle damage.

- Troponins need to be measured frequently in the immediate post-operative period. However, the 99th percentile of the upper reference limit, above which troponin levels become diagnostic of IPEMI and POMI, is still unknown.

- Coronary vasodilatation with glyceryl trinitrate (GTN) should not be suspended when indicated
- The early use of beta blocking drugs should be considered even with normal blood pressures and heart rates.
- If there is Unstable hemodynamic paramters
- Rapid diagnosis can be achieved by intraoperative Trans esophageal echocardiography IOTEEC.
- Coronary revascularization is urgent in this situation.

- Coronary angiography may not available, so revascularization depend on ITOEC and the preoperative coronary angiography for the anatomy of the ischemic part.

Local anesthetics toxicity

Local anesthetic toxicity can be seen in organs of the body that depend upon sodium channels for proper functioning. These include the central nervous system and heart. The CNS is more sensitive to the effects of local anesthetics than the cardiac system and will generally manifest signs/symptoms of toxicity first.

Esters	Max Dose (mg/kg)	Duration (h)
Chloroprocaine	12	0.5 − 1
Procaine	12	0.5 − 1
Cocaine	3	0.5 − 1
Tetracaine	3	1.5 − 6

Amides	Max Dose (mg/kg)	Duration (h)
Lidocaine	4.5/(7 with epi)	0.75 − 1.5
Mepivacaine	4.5/(7 with epi)	1 − 2
Prilocaine	8	0.5 − 1
Bupivacaine	3	1.5 − 8
Ropivacaine	3	1.5 − 8

Effects on Organ Systems

Central nervous system

The initial CNS symptoms are tinnitus, blurred vision, dizziness, tongue parathesias, and circumoral numbness.

Excitatory signs such as nervousness, agitation, restlessness, and muscle twitching are the result of blockade of inhibitory pathways.

Muscle twitching heralds the onset on tonic-clonic seizures.

The early signs/symptoms advance to CNS depression with slurred speech, drowsiness, unconsciousness, and then respiratory arrest. Patients who have received CNS depressant drugs may present with only CNS depression without any preceding excitatory signs.

Factors affecting the effects on the CNS

- Hypercarbia – Increased $PaCO_2$ lowers the seizure threshold with local anesthetic administration.

- There is a concomitant increase in cerebral blood flow which allows more local anesthetic to be delivered to the CNS.

- An increase in intracellular pH leads to ion-trapping of the local anesthetic.

- The acidosis caused by hypercarbia decreases the protein binding of local anesthetics making more drug available to the CNS.

- CNS Depression – Conscious patients receiving CNS depressant drugs such as benzodiazepines or IV anesthetic drugs will have higher seizure threshold, and may not

manifest seizure activity before complete CNS depression
results.

Cardiovascular system

Local anesthetics have directs effects on the heart and peripheral
blood vessels.

They block the fast sodium channels in the fast-conducting tissue of
Purkinje fibers and ventricles resulting in a decrease rate of
depolarization.

The effective refractory period and action potential duration are
also reduced by local anesthetics.

High concentrations can decrease conduction times leading to
prolonged PR intervals and widened QRS complexes, and even sinus
brady/arrest.

Ventricular arrhythmias, including fibrillation, are more likely to
occur with bupivacaine than lidocaine. Local anesthetics have a
dose-dependent negative inotropic effect.

This depressant effect is directly proportional to the drugs relative
potency . Patients with acidosis and/or hypoxia are at a greater risk
for the cardiac depressant effects of local anesthetics.

Cardiotoxicity of local anesthetics can be compared using the CC/CNS dose ratio that is the ratio of the dose causing cardiac collapse (CC) to the dose causing seizure/convulsions.

The lower the number the more cardiotoxic the drug (ex. The CC/CNS for bupivacaine is approximately 3 versus 7 for lidocaine).

It is important to note that patients under general anesthesia will typically present with cardiotoxicity as the first sign of local anesthetic toxicity.

Cardiovascular manifestations

- Chest pain
- Shortness of breath
- Palpitations
- Lightheadedness
- Diaphoresis
- Hypotension
- Syncope

Peripheral vascular effects

Low doses of local anesthetics may cause vasoconstriction, whereas, moderate or high doses result in vasodilation and decreased SVR. Cocaine is the only local anesthetic that causes vasoconstriction at all doses.

Different nerve blocks

The same amount of local anesthetic, serum levels are highest following intercostal blocks followed by epidural/caudal blocks, followed by brachial plexus and femoral/sciatic nerve blocks, followed by subcutaneous injections. This order parallels the vascular supply of each tissue. See Keyword below.

Absorption of Local Anesthetics (most to least)

- Intravenous

- Intercostal

- Caudal epidural

- Lumbar epidural

- Brachial plexus

- Subcutaneous

Pregnancy

Bupivacaine has been shown to have increased cardiotoxicity in pregnant women resulting in a decreased CC/CNS dose ration.

Methemoglobinemia

A side effect unique to prilocaine is methemoglobinemia at doses of at least 600mg. The liver metabolizes prilocaine to O-toluidine

which oxidizes hemoglobin to methaemoglobin.
Methemoglobinemia is readily treated with methylene blue

Clinical manifestations of methemoglobinemia

- Cyanosis
- Cutaneous discoloration (gray)
- Tachypnea
- Dyspnea
- Exercise intolerance
- Fatigue
- Dizziness and syncope
- Weakness

Treatement of local anesthetics toxicity

Prevention

Strict adherence to the guidelines of anesthetic dosing, identification of patients at increased risk, and implementation of appropriate anesthetic application techniques to avoid unintentional intravascular injection.

Airway compromise, significant hypotension, dysrhythmias, and seizures

Airway compromise

- Oxygenation by mask or nasal canula
- **Endotracheal intubation, and respiratory support by mechanical ventilation when needed.**

cardiovascular toxicity

- monitor the cardiovascular system
- intravenous fluids
- vasopressors as required. Small bolus doses of epinephrine are preferred. Vasopressin is not recommended
- CPR when cardiac arrest occurs.

Treatment of seizures

- Benzodiazepines are the drugs of choice for seizure control.
- Propofol can be used to control seizures but has the risk of potentiating cardiovascular toxicity.
- Refractory seizures may require neuromuscular blockade (e.g., with succinylcholine

Treatment of metabolic acidosis

- **By aggressive treatment of respiratory complications**
- **Correction of hypoxemia**
- **Correction of sever hypotension**
- **Consideration of sodium bicarbonate infusion**

Lipid emulsion

The intravenous (IV) infusion of lipid emulsions can reverse the cardiac and neurologic effects of local-anesthetic toxicity.

Allergic reactions due to local anesthetic toxicity

Can be treated with diphenhydramine or, for more serious reactions, epinephrine or corticosteroids

Methemoglobinemia should initially be treated symptomatically.

Subsequent treatment is guided by blood levels of methemoglobin; methylene blue and hyperbaric oxygen may be required in severe cases

Local ischemic or nerve toxicities

in the extremities with prolonged anesthesia or use of agents containing epinephrine.

Suspected nerve damage should prompt neurologic consultation for urgent peripheral nerve studies.

If vascular compromise, such as limb ischemia, is suspected, consult a vascular surgeon immediately. Therapy for extravasation (eg, warm compresses, phentolamine, nitroglycerin cream) should be initiated for localized vascular toxicity

References

1. College of Chest Physicians Antithrombotic T, Prevention of Thrombosis P: Executive summary: Antithrombotic Therapy and Prevention of Thrombosis, 9th ed: American College of Chest Physicians EvidenceBased Clinical Practice Guidelines. Chest 2012, 141(2 Suppl):7S–47S.

2. Pandey A, Patni N, Singh M, Guleria R: Assessment of risk and prophylaxis for deep vein thrombosis and pulmonary embolism in medically ill patients during their early days of hospital stay at a tertiary care center in a developing country. Vasc Health Risk Manag 2009, 5:643–648.

3. Naess IA, Christiansen SC, Romundstad P, Cannegieter SC, Rosendaal FR, Hammerstrom J: Incidence and mortality of venous thrombosis: a population-based study. J Thromb Haemost 2007, 5(4):692–699.

4. Fowkes FJ, Price JF, Fowkes FG: Incidence of diagnosed deep vein thrombosis in the general population: systematic review. Eur J Vasc Endovasc Surg 2003, 25(1):1–5

5. Cunningham RS: The role of low-molecular-weight heparins as supportive care therapy in cancer-associated thrombosis. Semin Oncol 2006, 33(2 Suppl 4):S17–25. quiz S41-12.

6. Alikhan R, Cohen AT, Combe S, Samama MM, Desjardins L, Eldor A, Janbon C, Leizorovicz A, Olsson CG, Turpie AG: Risk factors for venous thromboembolism in hospitalized patients with acute medical illness: analysis of the MEDENOX Study. Arch Intern Med 2004, 164(9):963–968.

7. Pomero F, Ageno W, Serraino C, Borretta V, Gianni M, Fenoglio L, Prisco D, Dentali F: The role of inherited thrombophilia in patients with isolated pulmonary embolism: A systematic review and a meta-analysis of the literature. Thromb Res 2014, 134(1):84–89.

8. Palkar AV, Karnik ND: Risk stratification, prevalence by hand-held microdoppler and in-hospital mortality of deep venous thrombosis in indoor geriatric population. J Assoc Physicians India 2013, 61(8):539–542.

9. Ho KM, Chavan S, Pilcher D: Omission of early thromboprophylaxis and mortality in critically ill patients: a multicenter registry study. Chest 2011, 140(6):1436–1446.

10. McLeod AG, Geerts W: Venous thromboembolism prophylaxis in critically ill patients. Crit Care Clin 2011, 27(4):765–780. v.

10. Xu XF, Yang YH, Zhai ZG, Liu S, Zhu GF, Li CS, Wang C: Prevalence and incidence of deep venous thrombosis among patients in medical intensive care unit. Zhonghua liu xing bing xue za zhi = Zhonghua liuxingbingxue zazhi 2008, 29(10):1034–1037.

11. 12.Spyropoulos AC, Anderson FA Jr, Fitzgerald G, Decousus H, Pini M, Chong BH, Zotz RB, Bergmann JF, Tapson V, Froehlich JB Monreal M, Merli GJ, Pavanello R, Turpie AG, Nakamura M, Piovella F, Kakkar AK, Spencer FA, IMPROVE Investigators: Predictive and associative models to identify hospitalized medical patients at risk for VTE. Chest 2011, 140(3):706–714.

12. Sud S, Mittmann N, Cook DJ, Geerts W, Chan B, Dodek P, Gould MK, Guyatt G, Arabi Y, Fowler RA: Screening and prevention of venous thromboembolism in critically ill patients: a decision analysis and economic evaluation. Am J Respir Crit Care Med 2011, 184(11):1289–1298.

13. Parikh KC, Oh D, Sittipunt C, Kalim H, Ullah S, Aggarwal SK: Venous thromboembolism prophylaxis in medical ICU patients in Asia (VOICE Asia): a multicenter, observational, cross-sectional study. Thromb Res 2012, 129(4):e152–158.

14. Samama MM, Dahl OE, Quinlan DJ, Mismetti P, Rosencher N: Quantification of risk factors for venous

15. Silliman CC. The two-event model of transfusion-related acute lung injury. CRIT CARE MED. 2006 May. 34(5 suppl):S124-31. [Medline].

16. Silliman CC, Curtis BR, Kopko PM, et al. Donor antibodies to HNA-3a implicated in TRALI reactions prime neutrophils and cause PMN-mediated damage to human pulmonary microvascular endothelial cells in a two-event in vitro model. BLOOD. 2007 Feb 15. 109(4):1752-5. [Medline].

17. Curtis BR, McFarland JG. Mechanisms of transfusion-related acute lung injury (TRALI): anti-leukocyte antibodies. CRIT CARE MED. 2006 May. 34(5 suppl):S118-23. [Medline].

18. Skeate RC, Eastlund T. Distinguishing between transfusion related acute lung injury and transfusion associated circulatory overload. CURR OPIN HEMATOL. 2007 Nov. 14(6):682-7. [Medline].

19. Garratty G. Immune hemolytic anemia associated with negative routine serology. SEMIN HEMATOL. 2005 Jul. 42(3):156-64. [Medline].

20. Capon SM, Goldfinger D. Acute hemolytic transfusion reaction, a paradigm of the systemic inflammatory response: new insights into pathophysiology and treatment. TRANSFUSION. 1995 Jun. 35(6):513-20.[Medline].

21. Davenport RD. The role of cytokines in hemolytic transfusion reactions. IMMUNOL INVEST. 1995 Jan-Feb. 24(1-2):319-31. [Medline].

22. Sandler SG, Berry E, Ziotnick A. Benign hemoglobinuria following transfusion of accidentally frozen blood.JAMA. 1976 Jun 28. 235(26):2850-1. [Medline].

23. Vamvakas EC, Pineda AA. Allergic and anaphylactic reactions. Popovsky MA, ed. TRANSFUSION REACTIONS. 2nd ed. Bethesda, Md: American Association of Blood Banks Press; 2001. 83-127.

24. Sandler SG, Mallory D, Malamut D, Eckrich R. IgA anaphylactic transfusion reactions. TRANSFUS MED REV. 1995 Jan. 9(1):1-8. [Medline]

25. Tinegate H, Birchall J, Gray A, Haggas R, Massey E, Norfolk D, et al. Guideline on the investigation and management of acute transfusion reactions Prepared by the BCSH Blood

Transfusion Task Force. BR J HAEMATOL. 2012 Oct. 159(2):143-53. [Medline].

26. Bluemle LW Jr. Hemolytic transfusion reactions causing acute renal failure. Serologic and clinical considerations. POSTGRAD MED. 1965 Nov. 38(5):484-9. [Medline].

27. Looney MR, Roubinian N, Gajic O, Gropper MA, Hubmayr RD, Lowell CA, et al. Prospective study on the clinical course and outcomes in transfusion-related acute lung injury*. CRIT CARE MED. 2014 Jul. 42(7):1676-87. [Medline].

28. Davenport RD. Pathophysiology of hemolytic transfusion reactions. SEMIN HEMATOL. 2005 Jul. 42(3):165-8.[Medline].

29. Kleinman S, Caulfield T, Chan P, et al. Toward an understanding of transfusion-related acute lung injury: statement of a consensus panel. TRANSFUSION. 2004 Dec. 44(12):1774-89. [Medline].

30. Ness PM, Shirey RS, Thoman SK, Buck SA. The differentiation of delayed serologic and delayed hemolytic transfusion reactions: incidence, long-term serologic findings, and clinical significance.TRANSFUSION. 1990 Oct. 30(8):688-93. [Medline].

31. Popovsky MA, Audet AM, Andrzejewski C Jr. Transfusion-associated circulatory overload in orthopedic surgery patients: a multi-institutional study. IMMUNOHEMATOLOGY. 1996. 12(2):87-9. [Medline].

32. Sanchez R, Toy P. Transfusion related acute lung injury: a pediatric perspective. PEDIATR BLOOD CANCER. 2005 Sep. 45(3):248-55. [Medline].

33. Sandler SG, Eckrich R, Malamut D, Mallory D. Hemagglutination assays for the diagnosis and prevention of IgA anaphylactic transfusion reactions. BLOOD. 1994 Sep 15. 84(6):2031-5. [Medline]. [Full Text].

34. Sazama K. Reports of 355 transfusion-associated deaths: 1976 through 1985. TRANSFUSION. 1990 Sep. 30(7):583-90. [Medline].

35. Sazama K, DeChristopher PJ, Dodd R, et al. Practice parameter for the recognition, management, and prevention of adverse consequences of blood transfusion. College of American Pathologists. ARCH PATHOL LAB MED. 2000 Jan. 124(1):61-70. [Medline].

36. Schmidt PJ. The mortality from incompatible transfusion. Sandler SG, Nusbacher J, Schanfield MS,

eds.IMMUNOBIOLOGY OF THE ERYTHROCYTE. New York, NY: Alan R. Liss and Co; 1980. 251-62.

37. Silliman CC, Ambruso DR, Boshkov LK. Transfusion-related acute lung injury. BLOOD. 2005 Mar 15. 105(6):2266-73. [Medline].

38. thromboembolism: a preliminary study for the development of a risk assessment tool. Haematologica 2003, 88(12):1410–1421.

39. Howell MD, Geraci JM, Knowlton AA: Congestive heart failure and outpatient risk of venous thromboembolism: a retrospective, case–control study. J Clin Epidemiol 2001, 54(8):810–816.

40. .Hull RD, Schellong SM, Tapson VF, Monreal M, Samama MM, Turpie AG, Wildgoose P, Yusen RD: Extended-duration thromboprophylaxis in acutely ill medical patients with recent reduced mobility: methodology for the EXCLAIM study. J Thromb Thrombolysis 2006, 22(1):31–38.

41. Knaus WA, Zimmerman JE, Wagner DP, Draper EA, Lawrence DE: APACHEacute physiology and chronic health evaluation: a physiologically based classification system. Crit Care Med 1981, 9(8):591–597.

42. Knaus WA, Draper EA, Wagner DP, Zimmerman JE: APACHE
    II: a severity of disease classification system. Crit Care Med
    1985, 13(10):818–829.

43. Markgraf R, Deutschinoff G, Pientka L, Scholten T, Lorenz C:
    Performance of the score systems Acute Physiology and
    Chronic Health Evaluation II and III at an interdisciplinary
    intensive care unit, after customization. Crit Care 2001,
    5(1):31–36.

44. Lawall H, Hoffmanns W, Hoffmanns P, Rapp U, Ames M, Pira
    A, Paar WD, Bramlage P, Diehm C: Prevalence of deep vein
    thrombosis (DVT) in non-surgical patients at hospital
    admission. Thromb Haemost 2007, 98(4):765–770.

45. Cheng G, Chan C, Liu YT, Choy YF, Wong MM, Yeung PK, Ng
    KL, Tsang LS, Wong RS: Incidence of Deep Vein Thrombosis
    in Hospitalized Chinese Medical Patients and the Impact of
    DVT Prophylaxis. Thrombosis 2011, 2011:629383.

46. Oger E, Bressollette L, Nonent M, Lacut K, Guias B,
    Couturaud F, Leroyer C, Mottier D: High prevalence of
    asymptomatic deep vein thrombosis on admission in a
    medical unit among elderly patients. Thromb Haemost 2002,
    88(4):592–597.

47. Crowther MA, Cook DJ: Thromboprophylaxis in medical-surgical critically ill patients. Curr Opin Crit Care 2008, 14(5):520–523. 25. Hirsch DR, Ingenito EP, Goldhaber SZ: Prevalence of deep venous thrombosis among patients in medical intensive care. JAMA 1995, 274(4):335–337.

48. Marik PE, Andrews L, Maini B: The incidence of deep venous thrombosis in ICU patients. Chest 1997, 111(3):661–664.

49. . Cook D, Douketis J, Meade M, Guyatt G, Zytaruk N, Granton J, Skrobik Y, Albert M, Fowler R, Hebert P, Pagliarello G, Friedrich J, Freitag A, Karachi T, Rabbat C, Heels-Ansdell D, Geerts W, Crowther M, Canadian Critical Care Trials Group:

50. Venous thromboembolism and bleeding in critically ill patients with severe renal insufficiency receiving dalteparin thromboprophylaxis:

51. Cook D, Crowther M, Meade M, Rabbat C, Griffith L, Schiff D, Geerts W, Guyatt G: Deep venous thrombosis in medical-surgical critically ill patients: prevalence, incidence, and risk factors. Crit Care Med 2005, 33(7):1565–1571.

52. PROTECT Investigators for the Canadian Critical Care Trials Group and the Australian and New Zealand Intensive Care Society Clinical Trials Group, Cook D, Meade M, Guyatt G, Walter S, Heels-Ansdell D, Warkentin TE, Zytaruk N, Crowther M, Geerts W, Cooper

53. DJ Vallance S, Qushmaq I, Rocha M, Berwanger O, Vlahakis NE: Dalteparin versus unfractionated heparin in critically ill patients. N Engl J Med 2011, 364(14):1305–1314.

54. Hong KC, Kim H, Kim JY, Kwak KS, Cho OM, Cha HY, Lim SH, Song YJ: Risk factors and incidence of deep vein thrombosis in lower extremities among critically ill patients. J Clin Nurs 2012, 21(13–14):1840–1846.

55. Wells PS: Integrated strategies for the diagnosis of venous thromboembolism. J Thromb Haemost 2007, 5(Suppl 1):41–50.

56. Tzoran I, Saharov G, Brenner B, Delsart D, Roman P, Visona A, Jimenez D, Monreal M: Silent pulmonary embolism in patients with proximal deep vein thrombosis in the lower limbs. J Thromb Haemost 2012, 10(4):564–571.

57. Li XY, Fan J, Cheng YQ, Wang Y, Yao C, Zhong NS: Incidence and prevention of venous thromboembolism in acutely ill hospitalized elderly Chinese. Chin Med J 2011, 124(3):335–340.

58. Berlot G, Calderan C, Vergolini A, Bianchi M, Viviani M, Bussani R, Torelli L, Lucangelo U: Pulmonary embolism in critically ill patients receiving antithrombotic prophylaxis: a clinical-pathologic studGuyton AC, Lindsey AW, Gilluly JJ. The limits of right ventricular compensation following acute increase in pulmonary circulatory resistance. Circ Res. 1954;2:326–32.

59. Molloy WD, Lee KY, Girling L, Schick U, Prewitt RM. Treatment of shock in a canine model of pulmonary embolism. Am Rev Respir Dis. 1984;130:870–4.

60. Szold O, Khoury W, Biderman P, Klausner JM, Halpern P, Weinbroum AA. Inhaled nitric oxide improves pulmonary functions following massive pulmonary embolism: a report of four patients and review of the literature. Lung. 2006;184:1–5.

61. Kjaergaard B, Rasmussen BS, de Neergaard S, Rasmussen LH, Kristensen SR. Extracorporeal cardiopulmonary support may be an efficient rescue of patients after massive pulmonary

62. embolism. An experimental porcine study. Thromb Res. 2012;129:e147–51.

63. Decousus H, Leizorovicz A, Parent F, Page Y, Tardy B, Girard P, Laporte S. A clinical trial of vena caval filters in prevention of pulmonary embolism in patients with proximal deep-vein thrombosis. Prevention du Risque d'Embolie Pulmonaire par Interruption Cave Study Group. N Engl J Med. 1998;338:409–15.View ArticlePubMed

64. Girard P, Meyer G, Parent F, Mismetti P. Medical literature, vena cava filters and evidence of efficacy. A descriptive review. Thromb Haemost. 2014;111:761–9.

65. PREPIC study group. Eight-year follow-up of patients with permanent vena cava filters in the prevention of pulmonary embolism: the PREPIC (Prevention du Risque d'Embolie Pulmonaire par Interruption Cave) randomized study. Circulation. 2005;112:416–22.

66. Thomas MJG, Gillon J, Desmond MJ. An organisers' view. Transfusion. 1996;36:626–627. [PubMed]

67. Network for the Advancement of Transfusion Alternatives. Transfusion medicine and alternatives to blood transfusion. Paris: R&J Éditions Médicales; 2000.

68. Spiess BD, Counts RB, Gould SA. Perioperative transfusion medicine. Baltimore, MD: Williams and Wilkins; 1998.

69. Forgie MA, Wells PS, Laupacis A, Fergusson D. Preoperative autologous donation decreases allogeneic transfusion but increases exposure to all red blood cell transfusion—results of a meta-analysis. Arch Intern Med. 1998;158:610–616. [PubMed]

70. Faught C, Wells P, Fergusson D, Laupacis A. Adverse effects of methods for minimizing perioperative allogeneic transfusion—a critical review of the literature. Transfus Med Rev. 1998;12:206–225. [PubMed]

71. Blumberg N, Heal JM. Transfusion immunomodulation. In: Anderson KC, Ness PM, editors. Scientific basis of transfusion medicine. 2nd ed. Philadelphia: W B Saunders; 2000. pp. 427–443.

72. Stein PD, Matta F, Hull RD. Increasing use of vena cava filters for prevention of pulmonary embolism. Am J Med. 2011;124:655–61.

73. Soriano SG, McManus ML, Sullivan LJ, Scott RM, Rockoff MA. Doppler sensory placement during neurosurgical procedures for children in prone position. J Neurosurg Anesthesiology. 1994;6:153–5.[PubMed]

74. Sounders JE. Pulmonary air embolism. J Clin Monit Comp. 2000;16:375–83. [PubMed]

75. Brechner TM, Brechner VL. An audible alarm for monitoring air embolism during neurosurgery. J Neurosurgery. 1977;47:201–4. [PubMed]

76. Stendel R, Gramm HJ, Schröder K, Lober C, Brock M. Transcranial doppler ultrasonography as a screening tool for detection of patent foramen ovale before surgery in sitting position. Anesthesiology.2000;93:971–5. [PubMed]

77. Valentino R, Hilbert G, Vargas F, Grison D. Computed tomographic scan of massive cerebral air embolism. Lancet. 2003;361:1848. [PubMed]

78. Takahashi T, Yano K, Kimura T, Komatsu T, Shimada Y. Prevention of venous air emboilsm by jugular venous compression Under superior sagital sinus pressure monitoring in bracycephalic patients during craniofacial reconstruction. Anesthesia. 1997;7:259–60. [PubMed]

79. Sibai AN, Baraka A, Moudawar A. Hazards of nitrous oxide administration in the presence of venous air embolism. Middle East J Anesthesiolo. 1996;13:259–71. [PubMed]

80. Archer DP, Pash MP, Mackie ME. Successful management of venous air embolism with ionotropic support. Neuroanesth Intensive care. 2001;48:204–8. [PubMed]

81. Durant TM, Long J. Pulmonary (venous) air embolism. Am Heart J. 1947;33:269–87. [PubMed]

82. Mehlhorn U, Burke EJ, Butler BD, Davis KL, Katz J, Melamed E, et al. Body position doesn't affect hemodynamic respond to venous air embolism in dogs. Anesth Analg. 1994;79:734–9. [PubMed]

83. Colley PS, Artu AA. Bunegin – albino catheter improves air retrieval and resuscitation from lethal air embolism in upright dogs. Anesth Analg. 1989;68:298–301. [PubMed]

84. Ericsson JA, Gottleb JD, Sweet RB. Close chest cardiac massage in the treatment of venous air embolism. N Eng J Med. 1964;270:1353–4. [PubMed]

85. Blanc P, Boussuges A, Henriette K, Sainty JM, Deleflie M. Iatrogenic cerebral air embolism, importance of an early hyperbaric oxygension. Intensive Care Med. 2002;28:559–63. [PubMed]

86. Dankner R, Gall N, Freidman G, Arad J. Recompression treatment of red sea diving accidents; a 23 years summary. Clin j Sport Med. 2005;15:253–6. [PubMed]

87. Ryu KH, Hindman BJ, Reasoner DK, Dexter F. Heparin reduces neurological impairment after cerebral arterial air embolism in rabbit. Stroke. 1996;27:303–10. [PubMed]

88. Dutka AJ, Mink RB, Pearson RR, Hollenbeck Effects of treatment with dexamethason on recovery from experimental cerebral air embolism. Under sea Biomed Res. 1992;19:131–41. [PubMed]

89. Mitchell SJ, pellet O, Gorman D. Cerebral protection by lidocain during cardiothoracic operations. Ann Thorac Surg. 1999;67:1117–24. [PubMed]

90. Ho A M, Ling E. Systemic air embolism after lung trauma. Anesthesiology. 1990;90:564–75. [PubMed]

91. Mam motto T, Hayashi Y, Obnishi Y, Kurno M. Incidence of venous and paradoxical air embolism in neurosurgical patients in sitting position; Detection by trasesophgeal

echocardiography. Acta Anesthesiolo Scand. 1998;42:643–5. [PubMed]

92. Fong J, Gadalla F, Druzin M. Venous air emboli occurring during cesarean section, the effect of patients' position. Can J Anesth. 1991;38:191–5. [PubMed]

93. Brouns R, De Surgeloose D, Neetens I, De Deyn PP. Fatal venous cerebral air embolism secondary to a disconnected central venous catheter. Cerebro Vasc Dis. 2006;21:212–4. [PubMed]

94. Dominique CM. Anesthesia for neurosurgery in sitting position; a case series. Anesth Intensive Care.2005;33:332–5. [PubMed]

95. Meyer PG, Cuttaree H, Charron B, Jarreau MM, Perie AC, Sainte-Rose C. Prevention of venous air embolism in pediatric neurosurgical procedures performed in sitting position by combined use of MAST suit and PEEP. Br J Anesth. 1994;73:795–800. [PubMed]

96. Kim TY, Rhee JE, Kim KS, Cha WC, Suh GJ, Jung SK. Etomidate should be used carefully for emergent

endotracheal intubation in patients with septic shock. J Korean Med Sci. 2008;23:988–991.[PMC free article] [PubMed]

97. Murray H, Marik PE. Etomidate for endotracheal intubation in sepsis: acknowledging the good while accepting the bad. Chest. 2005;127:707–709. [PubMed]

98. Arbous MS, Grobbee DE, van Kleef JW, de Lange JJ, Spoormans HH, Touw P, et al. Mortality associated with anaesthesia: a qualitative analysis to identify risk factors. Anaesthesia. 2001;56:1141–1153.[PubMed]

99. Merx MW, Weber C. Sepsis and the heart. Circulation. 2007;116:793–802. [PubMed]

100. Takaono M, Yogosawa T, Okawa-Takatsuji M, Aotsuka S. Effects of intravenous anesthetics on interleukin (IL)-6 and IL-10 production by lipopolysaccharide-stimulated mononuclear cells from healthy volunteers. Acta Anaesthesiol Scand. 2002;46:176–179. [PubMed]

101.   Kao SJ, Su CF, Liu DD, Chen HI. Endotoxin-induced acute lung injury and organ dysfunction are attenuated by pentobarbital anaesthesia. Clin Exp Pharmacol Physiol. 2007;34:480–487. [PubMed]

102.   Stowe DF, Bosnjak ZJ, Kampine JP. Comparison of etomidate, ketamine, midazolam, propofol, and thiopental on function and metabolism of isolated hearts. Anesth Analg. 1992;74:547–558. [PubMed]

103.   Kim SN, Son SC, Lee SM, Kim CS, Yoo DG, Lee SK, et al. Midazolam inhibits proinflammatory mediators in the lipopolysaccharide-activated macrophage. Anesthesiology. 2006;105:105–110. [PubMed]

104.   Shafer A. Complications of sedation with midazolam in the intensive care unit and a comparison with other sedative regimens. Crit Care Med. 1998;26:947–956. [PubMed]

105.   Pichot C, Geloen A, Ghignone M, Quintin L. Alpha-2 agonists to reduce vasopressor requirements in septic shock? Med Hypotheses. 2010;75:652–656. [PubMed]

106.   . Pandharipande PP, Sanders RD, Girard TD, McGrane S, Thompson JL, Shintani AK, et al. Effect of dexmedetomidine versus lorazepam on outcome in patients with sepsis: an a priori-designed analysis of the MENDS randomized controlled trial. Crit Care. 2010;14:R38. [PMC free article] [PubMed]

107.   Taniguchi T, Kidani Y, Kanakura H, Takemoto Y, Yamamoto K. Effects of dexmedetomidine on mortality rate and inflammatory responses to endotoxin-induced shock in rats. Crit Care Med. 2004;32:1322–1326. [PubMed]

108.   Vincent JL, Weil MH. Fluid challenge revisited. Crit Care Med. 2006;34:1333–1337. [PubMed]

109.   Rivers E, Nguyen B, Havstad S, Ressler J, Muzzin A, Knoblich B, et al. Early goal-directed therapy in the treatment of severe sepsis and septic shock. N Engl J Med. 2001;345:1368–1377. [PubMed]

110.   Hollenberg SM, Ahrens TS, Annane D, Astiz ME, Chalfin DB, Dasta JF, et al. Practice parameters for hemodynamic support of sepsis in adult patients: 2004 update. Crit Care Med. 2004;32:1928–1948. [PubMed]

111.   Michard F, Teboul JL. Predicting fluid responsiveness in ICU patients: a critical analysis of the evidence.Chest. 2002;121:2000–2008. [PubMed]

112.   Antonelli M, Levy M, Andrews PJ, Chastre J, Hudson
LD, Manthous C, et al. Hemodynamic monitoring in shock
and implications for management. International Consensus
Conference, Paris, France, 27-28 April 2006. Intensive Care
Med. 2007;33:575–590. [PubMed]

113.   Vieillard-Baron A, Chergui K, Rabiller A, Peyrouset O,
Page B, Beauchet A, et al. Superior vena caval collapsibility
as a gauge of volume status in ventilated septic
patients. Intensive Care Med. 2004;30:1734–
1739. [PubMed]

114.   Dellinger RP, Levy MM, Carlet JM, Bion J, Parker MM,
Jaeschke R, et al. Surviving Sepsis Campaign: international
guidelines for management of severe sepsis and septic
shock: 2008. Crit Care Med.2008;36:296–327. [PubMed]

115.   . Leone M, Bourgoin A, Cambon S, Dubuc M,
Albanese J, Martin C. Empirical antimicrobial therapy of
septic shock patients: adequacy and impact on the
outcome. Crit Care Med. 2003;31:462–467. [PubMed]

116.   Tsuneyoshi I, Yamada H, Kakihana Y, Nakamura M,
Nakano Y, Boyle WA., 3rd Hemodynamic and metabolic
effects of low-dose vasopressin infusions in vasodilatory
septic shock. Crit Care Med.2001;29:487–493. [PubMed]

117.   Beale RJ, Hollenberg SM, Vincent JL, Parrillo JE. Vasopressor and inotropic support in septic shock: an evidence-based review. Crit Care Med. 2004;32(11 Suppl):S455–S465. [PubMed]

118.   . Fisher MM, Doig GS. Prevention of anaphylactic reactions to anaesthetic drugs. Drug Saf. 2004;27:393–410. [PubMed]

119.   Naguib M, Magboul MM. Adverse effects of neuromuscular blockers and their antagonists. Drug Saf.1998;18:99–116. [PubMed]

120.   Baldo BA, Fisher MM. Substituted ammonium ions as allergenic determinants in drug allergy. Nature.1983;306:262–4. [PubMed]

121.   Didier A, Cador D, Bongrand P, Furstoss R, Fourneron P, Senft M, et al. Role of the quaternary ammonium ion determinants in allergy to muscle relaxants. J Allergy Clin Immunol. 1987;79:578–84.[PubMed]

122.   Marone G, Stellato C. Activation of human mast cells and basophils by general anaesthetic drugs.Monogr Allergy. 1992;30:54–73. [PubMed]

123.   Naguib M, Samarkandi AH, Bakhamees HS, Magboul MA, el Bakry AK. Histamine-release haemodynamic changes produced by rocuronium, vecuronium, mivacurium, atracurium and tubocurarine. Br J Anaesth. 1995;75:588–92. [PubMed]

124.   Koppert W, Blunk JA, Petersen LJ, Skov P, Rentsch K, Schmelz M. Different patterns of mast cell activation by muscle relaxants in humaskin. Anesthesiology. 2001;95:659–67. [PubMed]

125.   Ebo DG, Stevens WJ. IGE-mediated natural rubber latex allergy: An update. Acta Clin Belg.2002;57:58–70. [PubMed]

126.   Baldo BA, Fisher MM. Mechanisms in IgE-dependent anaphylaxis to anesthetic drugs. Ann Fr Anesth Reanim. 1993;12:131–40. [PubMed]

127.   Leynadier F, Sansarricq M, Didier JM, Dry J. Prick tests in the diagnosis of anaphylaxis to general anaesthetics. Br J Anaesth. 1987;59:683–9. [PubMed]

128.   Ricci G, Gentili A, Di Lorenzo F, Righetti F, Pigna A, Masi M, et al. Latex allergy in subjects who had undergone multiple surgical procedures for bladder exstrophy: Relationship with clinical intervention and atopic diseases. BJU Int. 1999;84:1058–62. [PubMed]

129. Sussman GL, Beezhold DH, Kurup VP. Allergens and natural rubber proteins. J Allergy Clin Immunol.2002;110:S33–9. [PubMed]

130. Cogen FC, Beezhold DH. Hair glue anaphylaxis: A hidden latex allergy. Ann Allergy Asthma Immunol.2002;88:61–3. [PubMed]

131. Hepner DL, Castells MC. Latex allergy: An update. Anesth Analg. 2003;96:1219–29. [PubMed]

132. Turjanmaa K, Reunala T, Tuimala R, Karkkainen T. Severe IgE-mediated allergy to surgical gloves.Allergy. 1984;2:S35.

133. Ewan PW, Dugué P, Mirakian R, Dixon TA, Harper JN, Nasser SM. BSACI guidelines for the investigation of suspected anaphylaxis during general anaesthesia. Clin Exp Allergy. 2010;40:15–31.[PubMed]

134. Alenius H, Kurup V, Kelly K, Palosuo T, Turjanmaa K, Fink J. Latex allergy: Frequent occurrence of IgE antibodies to a cluster of 11 latex proteins in patients with spina bifida and histories of anaphylaxis. J Lab Clin Med. 1994;123:712–20. [PubMed]

135. methods. Allerg Immunol (Paris) 2006;38:24–30. [PubMed]

136.   Levy J. Common anaphylactic and anaphylactoid reactions. In: Levy J, editor. Anaphylactic Reactions in Anesthesia and Intensive Care. Boston: Butterworth-Heinemann; 1992. p. 83.

137.   Salkind AR, Cuddy PG, Foxworth JW. Is this patient allergic to penicillin? An evidence-based analysis of the likelihood of penicillin allergy. JAMA. 2001;285:2498–505. [PubMed]

138.   Anne S, Reisman RE. Risk of administering cephalosporin antibiotics to patients with histories of penicillin allergy. Ann Allergy Asthma Immunol. 1995;74:167–70. [PubMed]

139.   Kelkar PS, Li JTC. Cephalosporin allergy. N Engl J Med. 2001;345:804–9. [PubMed]

140.   Cook FV, Farrar WE., Jr Vancomycin revisited. Ann Intern Med. 1978;88:813–8. [PubMed]

141.   Park M, Markus P, Matesic D, Li JT. Safety and effectiveness of a preoperative allergy clinic in decreasing vancomycin use in patients with a history of penicillin allergy. Ann Allergy Asthma Immunol.2006;97:681–7. [PubMed]

142.   Newfield P, Roizen MF. Hazards of rapid administration of vancomycin. Ann Intern Med. 1979;91:581.[PubMed]

143.   Renz CL, Laroche D, Thurn JD, Finn HA, Lynch JP, Thisted R, et al. Tryptase levels are not increased during vancomycin-inducedanaphylactoid reactions. Anesthesiology. 1998;89:620–5. [PubMed]

144.   Vervloet D, Pradal M, Castelain M. 2nd ed. Uppsala, Sweden: Pharmacia and Upjohn; 1999. Drug allergy.

145.   Harboe T, Guttormsen AB, Irgens A, Dybendal T, Florvaag E. Anaphylaxis during anesthesia in Norway: A 6-year single-center follow-up study. Anesthesiology. 2005;102:897–903. [PubMed]

146.   Ring J. Anaphylactoid reactions to intravenous solutions used for volume substitution. Clin Rev Allergy.1991;9:397–414. [PubMed]

147.   Ring J. Anaphylactoid reactions to plasma substitutes. Int Anesthesiol Clin. 1985;23:67–95. [PubMed]

148.   Laxenaire MC, Charpentier C, Feldman L. Anaphylactoid reactions to colloid plasma substitutes: Incidence, risk factors, and mechanisms–A French multicenter prospective study [in French] Ann Fr Anesth Reanim. 1994;13:301–10. [PubMed]

149.   Mertes PM, Moneret-Vautrin DA, Leynadier F, Laxenaire MC. Skin reactions to intradermal neuromuscular blocking agent injections: a randomized multicenter trial in healthy volunteers. Anesthesiology. Aug 2007;107(2):245-252. 27. Fisher MM. The preoperative detection of risk of anaphylaxis during anaesthesia. Anaesth Intensive Care. Dec 2007;35(6):899-902. 28.

150.   Ebo DG, Bridts CH, Hagendorens MM, Aerts NE, De Clerck LS, Stevens WJ. Basophil activation test by flow cytometry: Present and future applications in allergology. Cytometry B Clin Cytom. Apr 15 2008;74B(4):201-210.

151.   Laroche D, Lefrancois C, Gerard JL, et al. Early diagnosis of anaphylactic reactions to neuromuscular blocking drugs. Br J Anaesth. 1992;69(6):611-614.

152.   Guttormsen AB, Johansson SG, Oman H, Wilhelmsen V, Nopp A. No consumption of IgE antibody in serum during allergic drug anaphylaxis. Allergy. Nov 2007;62(11):1326-1330.

153.   Mertes PM, Laxenaire MC. Allergy and anaphylaxis in anaesthesia. Minerva Anestesiol. May 2004;70(5):285-291.

154.   Baumann A, Studnicska D, Audibert G, et al. Refractory anaphylactic cardiac arrest after succinylcholine administration. Anesth Analg. Jul 2009;109(1):137-140.

155.   Kroigaard M, Garvey LH, Menne T, Husum B. Allergic reactions in anaesthesia: are suspected causes confirmed on subsequent testing? Br J Anaesth. Oct 2005;95(4):468-471.

156.   Laxenaire MC, Mouton C, Frederic A, Viry-Babel F, Bouchon Y. Anaphylactic shock after tourniquet removal in orthopedic surgery. Ann Fr Anesth Reanim. 1996;15(2):179-184.

157.   Laroche D, Dubois F, Gérard J, Lefrançois C, André B, Vergnaud M. Radioimmunoassy for plasma histamine : a study of false positive and false negative values. Br J Anaesth. 1995;74:430- 437.

158.   Fisher MM, Baldo BA. Mast cell tryptase in anaesthetic anaphylactoid reactions. Br J Anaesth. Jan 1998;80(1):26-29.

159.   Malinovsky JM, Decagny S, Wessel F, Guilloux L, Mertes PM. Systematic follow-up increases incidence of anaphylaxis during adverse reactions in anesthetized patients. Acta Anaesthesiol Scand. Feb 2008;52(2):175-181.

160.   Baldo BA, Fisher MM. Anaphylaxis to muscle relaxant drugs: cross-reactivity and molecular basis of binding of IgE antibodies detected by radioimmunoassay. Mol Immunol. Dec 1983;20(12):1393-1400.

161.   Fisher MM, Baldo BA. Immunoassays in the diagnosis of anaphylaxis to neuromuscular blocking drugs : the value of morphine for the detection of IgE antibodies in allergic subjects. Anaesth Intensive Care. 2000;28:167-170.

162.   Gueant JL, Mata E, Monin B, et al. Evaluation of a new reactive solid phase for radioimmunoassay of serum specific IgE against muscle relaxant drugs. Allergy. 1991;46(6):452- 458.

163.   Guilloux L, Ricard-Blum S, Ville G, Motin J. A new radioimmunoassay using a commercially available solid support for the detection of IgE antibodies against muscle relaxants. J Allergy Clin Immunol. 1992;90(2):153-159.

164.   Ebo DG, Venemalm L, Bridts CH, et al. Immunoglobulin E antibodies to rocuronium: a new diagnostic tool. Anesthesiology. Aug 2007;107(2):253-259.

165.   Baldo BA, Fisher MM, Harle DG. Allergy to thiopentone. Clin Rev Allergy. 1991;9(3-4):295- 308

166.   Fisher MM, Harle DG, Baldo BA. Anaphylactoid reactions to narcotic analgesics. Clin Rev Allergy. 1991;9(3-4):309-31

167.   Gueant JL, Mata E, Masson C, et al. Non-specific cross-reactivity of hydrophobic serum IgE to hydrophobic drugs. Mol Immunol. Mar 1995;32(4):259-266. Perioperative Anaphylaxis 168

168.	Hemery ML, Arnoux B, Rongier M, Barbotte E, Bousquet J, Demoly P. Correlation between former and new assays of latex IgE-specific determination using the K82 and K82 recombinant allergens from the Pharmacia Diagnostics laboratory. Allergy. Jan 2005;60(1):131-132.

169.	Soetens FM. Anaphylaxis during anaesthesia: diagnosis and treatment. Acta Anaesthesiol Belg. 2004;55(3):229-237. 50. Fisher MM, Merefield D, Baldo B. Failure to prevent an anaphylactic reaction to a second neuromuscular blocking drug during anaesthesia. Br J Anaesth. 1999;82(5):770-773

170.	Levy JH, Gottge M, Szlam F, Zaffer R, McCall C. Weal and flare responses to intradermal rocuronium and cisatracurium in humans. Br J Anaesth. 2000;85:844-849.

171.	Berg CM, Heier T, Wilhelmsen V, Florvaag E. Rocuronium and cisatracurium-positive skin tests in non-allergic volunteers: determination of drug concentration thresholds using a dilution titration technique. Acta Anaesthesiol Scand. 2003;47(5):576-582.

172.	Mertes PM, Laxenaire M. Anaphylaxis during general anaesthesia. Prevention and management. CNS Drugs. 2000;14(2):115-133

173.   Thacker MA, Davis FM. Subsequent general anaesthesia in patients with a history of previous anaphylactoid/anaphylactic reaction to muscle relaxant. Anaesth Intensive Care. 1999;27(2):190- 193.

174.   Laxenaire MC, Moneret-Vautrin DA. Allergy and anaesthesia. Current Opinion in anaesthesiology. 1992;5:436-441.

175.   Leynadier F, Sansarricq M, Didier JM, Dry J. Prick tests in the diagnosis of anaphylaxis to general anaesthetics. Br J Anaesth. 1987;59(6):683-689.

176.   Fisher MM, Bowey CJ. Intradermal compared with prick testing in the diagnosis of anaesthetic allergy. Br J Anaesth. 1997;79(1):59-63.

177.   McKinnon RP. Allergic reactions during anaesthesia. Curr Op Anaesth. 1996;9:267-270. 59. Blanca M, Romano A, Torres MJ, et al. Update on the evaluation of hypersensitivity reactions to betalactams. Allergy. Feb 2009;64(2):183-193

178.   Turjanmaa K, Palosuo T, Alenius H, et al. Latex allergy diagnosis: in vivo and in vitro standardization of a natural rubber latex extract. Allergy. 1997;52(1):41-50.

179.   Mertes PM, Malinovsky JM, Mouton-Faivre C, et al. Anaphylaxis to dyes during the perioperative period: reports of 14 clinical cases. J Allergy Clin Immunol. Aug 2008;122(2):348- 352. 63.

180.   Mata E, Gueant JL, Moneret-Vautrin DA, et al. Clinical evaluation of in vitro leukocyte histamine release in allergy to muscle relaxant drugs. Allergy. 1992;47(5):471-476. 64.

181.   Assem E. Release of eosinophil cationic protein (ECP) in anaphylactoid anaesthetic reactions in vivo and in vitro. Agents Actions. 1994;41:C11-C13.

182.   Assem E. Leukotriene C4 release from blood cells in vitro in patients with anaphylactoid reactions to neuromuscular blockers. Agents Actions. 1993;38:C242-C244

183.   Abuaf N, Rajoely B, Ghazouani E, et al. Validation of a flow cytometric assay detecting in vitro basophil activation for the diagnosis of muscle relaxant allergy. J Allergy Clin Immunol. 1999;104(2 Pt 1):411-418.

184.   Sabbah A, Drouet M, Sainte-Laudry J, Lauret MG, Loiry M. [Contribution of flow cytometry to allergologic diagnosis]. Allerg Immunol (Paris). Jan 1997;29(1):15-21.

185.   Sainte-Laudy J, Vallon C, Guerin JC. Analysis of membrane expression of the CD63 human basophil activation marker. Applications to allergologic diagnosis. Allerg Immunol (Paris). 1994;26(6):211-214.

186.   Monneret G, Benoit Y, Gutowski M, Bienvenu J. Detection of basophil activation by flow cytométrie in patients with allergy to muscle-relaxant drugs. Anesthesiology. 2000;92(1):275-

187.   Bousquet PJ, Pipet A, Bousquet-Rouanet L, Demoly P. Oral challenges are needed in the diagnosis of beta-lactam hypersensitivity. Clin Exp Allergy. Jan 2008;38(1):185-190.

188.   Demoly P, Romano A, Botelho C, et al. Determining the negative predictive value of provocation tests with beta-lactams. Allergy. Oct 26 2009.

189.   Fisher MM, Bowey CJ. Alleged allergy to local anaesthetics. Anaesth Intensive Care. Dec 1997;25(6):611-614.

190.   Florvaag E, Johansson SG, Oman H, et al. Prevalence of IgE antibodies to morphine. Relation to the high and low incidences of NMBA anaphylaxis in Norway and Sweden, respectively. Acta Anaesthesiol Scand. Apr 2005;49(4):437-444.

191.   Garvey LH, Roed-Petersen J, Menne T, Husum B. Danish Anaesthesia Allergy Centre - preliminary results. Acta Anaesthesiol Scand. Nov 2001;45(10):1204-1209.

192.   Bhananker SM, O'Donnell JT, Salemi JR, Bishop MJ. The risk of anaphylactic reactions to rocuronium in the United States is comparable to that of vecuronium: an analysis of food and drug administration reporting of adverse events. Anesth Analg. Sep 2005;101(3):819-822, table of contents. 80. Galletly DC, Treuren BC. Anaphylactoid reactions during anaesthesia. Seven years' experience of intradermal testing. Anaesthesia. 1985;40(4):329-333.

193.   Heier T, Guttormsen AB. Anaphylactic reactions during induction of anaesthesia using rocuronium for muscle relaxation: a report including 3 cases. Acta Anaesthesiol Scand. Aug 2000;44(7):775-781.

194.   Florvaag E, Johansson SG. The pholcodine story. Immunol Allergy Clin North Am. Aug 2009;29(3):419-427.

195.   Gueant JL, Gueant-Rodriguez RM, Cornejo-Garcia JA, Viola M, Blanca M, Romano A. Gene variants of IL13, IL4, and IL4RA are predictors of beta-lactam allergy. J Allergy Clin Immunol. Feb 2009;123(2):509; author reply 509-510.

196.   Birnbaum J, Vervloet D. Allergy to muscle relaxants. Clin Rev Allergy. 1991;9(3-4):281-293.

197. . Harboe T, Johansson SG, Florvaag E, Oman H. Pholcodine exposure raises serum IgE in patients with previous anaphylaxis to neuromuscular blocking agents. Allergy. Dec 2007;62(12):1445- 1450.

198. Johansson SG, Florvaag E, Oman H, et al. National pholcodine consumption and prevalence of IgE-sensitization: a multicentre study. Allergy. Oct 1 2009.

199. Doenicke AW, Czeslick E, Moss J, Hoernecke R. Onset time, endotracheal intubating conditions, and plasma histamine after cisatracurium and vecuronium administration. Anesth Analg. Aug 1998;87(2):434-438.

200. Jooste E, Klafter F, Hirshman CA, Emala CW. A mechanism for rapacuronium-induced bronchospasm: M2 muscarinic receptor antagonism. Anesthesiology. 2003;98(4):906-911

201. Thygesen K, Alpert JS, White HD Joint ESC/ACCF/AHA/WHF Task Force for the Redefinition of Myocardial Infarction. Universal definition of myocardial infarction. Eur Heart J 2007;**28**:2525-2538.

202. Auerbach A, Goldman LAssessing and reducing the cardiac risk of noncardiac surgery. Circulation2006;**113**:1361-1376.

203.   Brilakis E, Banerjee S, Berger P Perioperative management of patients with coronary stents. J Am Coll Cardiol2007;**49**:2145-2150.

204.   Cohen MC, Aretz T Histological analysis of coronary artery in fatal postoperative myocardial infarction.Cardiovasc Pathol 1999;**8**:133-139.

205.   Goldfrank LR, Flomenbaum NE, Lewin NA, et al. 1507-17. GOLDFRANK'S TOXICOLOGIC EMERGENCIES. 6th ed. New York: McGraw-Hill; 1998. 897-903. 2003 Jun. 17(3):357-8. [Medline].

206.   [Guideline] The Association of Anaesthetists of Great Britain and Ireland. Guidelines for the Management of Severe Local Anaesthetic Toxicity. 2007. [Full Text].

207.   Leskiw U, Weinberg GL. Lipid resuscitation for local anesthetic toxicity: is it really lifesaving?. CURR OPIN ANAESTHESIOL. 2009 Oct. 22(5):667-71. [Medline].

208.   Weinberg G, Ripper R, Feinstein DL, Hoffman W. Lipid emulsion infusion rescues dogs from bupivacaine-induced cardiac toxicity. REG ANESTH PAIN MED. 2003 May-Jun. 28(3):198-202. [Medline].

209.   Rosenblatt MA, Abel M, Fischer GW, Itzkovich CJ, Eisenkraft JB. Successful use of a 20% lipid emulsion to

resuscitate a patient after a presumed bupivacaine-related cardiac arrest. ANESTHESIOLOGY. 2006 Jul. 105(1):217-8. [Medline].

210.   Litz RJ, Roessel T, Heller AR, Stehr SN. Reversal of central nervous system and cardiac toxicity after local anesthetic intoxication by lipid emulsion injection. ANESTH ANALG. 2008 May. 106(5):1575-7, table of contents. [Medline].

211.   Litz RJ, Popp M, Stehr SN, Koch T. Successful resuscitation of a patient with ropivacaine-induced asystole after axillary plexus block using lipid infusion. ANAESTHESIA. 2006 Aug. 61(8):800-1. [Medline].

212.   Foxall G, McCahon R, Lamb J, Hardman JG, Bedforth NM. Levobupivacaine-induced seizures and cardiovascular collapse treated with Intralipid. ANAESTHESIA. 2007 May. 62(5):516-8. [Medline].

213.   Zimmer C, Piepenbrink K, Riest G, Peters J. [Cardiotoxic and neurotoxic effects after accidental intravascular bupivacaine administration. Therapy with lidocaine propofol and lipid emulsion]. ANAESTHESIST. 2007 May. 56(5):449-53. [Medline].

214.   Ludot H, Tharin JY, Belouadah M, Mazoit JX, Malinovsky JM. Successful resuscitation after ropivacaine and lidocaine-induced ventricular arrhythmia following posterior lumbar plexus block in a child. ANESTH ANALG. 2008 May. 106(5):1572-4, table of contents. [Medline]. [Full Text].

215.   Warren JA, Thoma RB, Georgescu A, Shah SJ. Intravenous lipid infusion in the successful resuscitation of local anesthetic-induced cardiovascular collapse after supraclavicular brachial plexus block. ANESTH ANALG. 2008 May. 106(5):1578-80, table of contents. [Medline]. [Full Text].

216.   Marwick PC, Levin AI, Coetzee AR. Recurrence of cardiotoxicity after lipid rescue from bupivacaine-induced cardiac arrest. ANESTH ANALG. 2009 Apr. 108(4):1344-6. [Medline]. [Full Text].

217.   Weinberg GL, Di Gregorio G, Ripper R, et al. Resuscitation with lipid versus epinephrine in a rat model of bupivacaine overdose. ANESTHESIOLOGY. 2008 May. 108(5):907-13. [Medline].

218.   Di Gregorio G, Schwartz D, Ripper R, et al. Lipid emulsion is superior to vasopressin in a rodent model of

resuscitation from toxin-induced cardiac arrest. CRIT CARE MED. 2009 Mar. 37(3):993-9. [Medline].

219.   Mayr VD, Mitterschiffthaler L, Neurauter A, et al. A comparison of the combination of epinephrine and vasopressin with lipid emulsion in a porcine model of asphyxial cardiac arrest after intravenous injection of bupivacaine. ANESTH ANALG. 2008 May. 106(5):1566-71, table of contents. [Medline].

220.   Harvey M, Cave G, Kazemi A. Intralipid infusion diminishes return of spontaneous circulation after hypoxic cardiac arrest in rabbits. ANESTH ANALG. 2009 Apr. 108(4):1163-8. [Medline].

221.   Weinberg G. LipidRescue: resuscitation for cardiac toxicity. Available at http://www.lipidrescue.org/.

222.   Resuscitation Council (UK). Cardiac arrest or cardiovascular collapse caused by local anaesthetic. Available at http://www.resus.org.uk/pages/caLocalA.htm. Accessed: July 2008.

223.   Hiller DB, Gregorio GD, Ripper R, Kelly K, Massad M, Edelman L, et al. Epinephrine impairs lipid resuscitation from bupivacaine overdose: a threshold effect. ANESTHESIOLOGY. 2009 Sep. 111(3):498-505.[Medline].

www.ingramcontent.com/pod-product-compliance
Lightning Source LLC
Chambersburg PA
CBHW070258190526
45169CB00001B/465